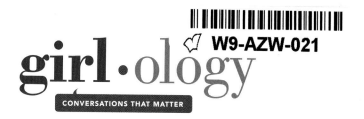

girl·ology
CONVERSATIONS THAT MATTER

W9-AZW-021

THERE'S SOMETHING NEW ABOUT YOU

A girl's guide to growing up

BY: MELISA HOLMES, M.D. & TRISH HUTCHISON, M.D.

3LEAF Press

Charleston, South Carolina

Library of Congress Cataloging-in-Publication Data

Holmes, Melisa.

Girlology's There's Something New About You: A Girl's Guide to Growing Up / Melisa Holmes, M.D., Trish Hutchison, M.D.

ISBN-13: 978-1-939433-33-6

Publisher: 3 LEAF Press
                P. O. Box 1419
                Mt. Pleasant, SC 29465

Illustrations by Lisa Perrett
Cover design by Ashley Inzer
Girls' short stories by Barbara Robertson

Contents

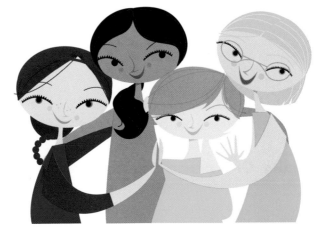

A Message to Parents

If you're flipping through this book, you must have been asked one of "those" questions recently. Or maybe you were surprised to hear your little girl having girl talk that sounded like big-girl talk. Perhaps you've noticed your daughter or one of her friends showing signs of puberty, and you realize it's time for that talk.

That's why we're here.

Since 2002, *Girlology* has been helping families improve communication about puberty, sexuality, and adolescent behaviors. This book is based on our most popular daughter-mom program: "Something New About You." It is written for girls ages eight through twelve, and it covers everything about puberty without diving into reproduction and its associated topics. Like many books, it's most helpful to your girl when she has an adult to follow along and answer questions or hear her comments.

There are several reasons to share a book like this with your elementary-age girl. Obviously, you want her to be prepared for the changes that come with puberty, and whether you're ready or not, puberty sneaks in as early as age seven. You want her to have an accurate and trusted source for information rather than relying on the tales she hears on the playground from some kid who has been miseducated by an older sibling. But most important, you want to establish yourself as her "go to" person when it comes to health and sexuality education. You do. Really. Open communication about these topics has been shown to delay the onset of sexual behaviors and to improve protective behaviors among teens. And now is the ideal time to open those communication lines.

Scared? Don't be. It's a lot easier than you think. And besides, we promise to offer help along the way. Visit our website at www.girlology.com for talking tips and other resources. You can also turn to the next books in our series: *Girlology: A Girl's Guide to Stuff That Matters*, and for high school and college girls, *Girlology's Hang Ups, Hook Ups, and Holding Out*.

Get started on those conversations that matter!

Melisa Holmes, M.D.
Trish Hutchison, M.D.
Girlology

CHAPTER 1

Something New

Claire

LILY IS MY BEST FRIEND in the whole world. We've
known each other since we were three—almost nine years.
She is pretty and smart and nice. We do everything together.
We have always done everything together. When Lily learned
to swim, I learned to swim. When Lily took ballet lessons,
I took ballet. When Lily took horseback riding lessons, I did,
too. Although she was always a little more graceful and a little
better at everything than me, it never seemed to matter.
I would try harder and I could hang in there. If I put my mind
to it, I could do what she did.

   We tell each other everything. We have no secrets. We
know the names of each other's secret crushes. We tell each
other every little embarrassing thing that happens. She is the

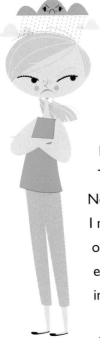

one person that knows me better than anyone else. I have always loved my friend Lily. Actually *everybody* loves Lily. But today, if I hear the name Lily, I will scream! I will scream so loud it will shatter a window. If I think about my best friend, I will get so angry, I will throw something. The thing is, she hasn't done anything to me. Nothing. Nada. Zip. She's always super nice. I mean, if you knew her, you would totally be on her side. But it's just not fair! Everything is easy for her. Did I mention that she is perfect in every way?

Nothing is easy for me. I am too small, too skinny, and not too great at math. My mother says, "Claire, you are the perfect you. You *are* beautiful and smart." Well, duh, she's like my mom. What else is she going to say? But she's wrong. All of my friends are looking older. They are "developing" as Ms. Schwartz, our science teacher, says. Me? I could still pass for a seven-year-old! What if I am some sort of freak that never develops?

Lily just called me. From her new cell phone! I try to be excited for her. Listening to her happy, squeaking voice, I forget about how frustrated I am and how perfect she is. Still, I am now officially the last girl I know who doesn't have a cell phone. My mother says that I am too young for one. She doesn't understand why I would need a phone. Once again,

she thinks that I am just a kid. She thinks
that because I am small, I am too little
to be taken seriously. Well, my mother
seriously makes me a *little* crazy!

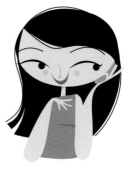

Does the word " puberty " make you want to
roll your eyes? Does it sound like some grown-up word
that comes before a very embarrassing talk? Puberty can be confusing, embarrassing, and exciting all at once. That's the way it is
for almost everyone. Reading a book about it may seem really
awkward or really helpful, or maybe a little of both.

The more you learn about your body and the way it works,
the less embarrassing it will be. It's even pretty interesting sometimes, and you'll be glad you know what's going on. Even though
you will be reading about some awkward stuff, like breasts growing, pubic hairs sprouting, acne blooming, and periods starting,
you'll find it less embarrassing as you learn more. You may think
some of what you learn here is gross, some of it is neat, and some
of it . . . well, you may not really know what to think about some
of it. That's all normal! We'll teach you some things that will
make puberty easier to understand and easier to talk about. We
promise you three things by the end of this book:

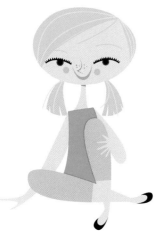

1. You'll be proud you know so much.

2. You will be more comfortable asking questions about growing up.

3. You will be more comfortable talking about your body and the amazing (and sometimes confusing) things it does.

What Is Puberty, Anyway?

Puberty is a pretty unusual word. What exactly does it mean? Well, the word "puberty" comes from a Latin word, *pubertas*, which means "adulthood." It also comes from another Latin word, *pubescere*, which means "to grow hairy or mossy." Hmmm. That's pretty descriptive.

To say it simply, puberty is the process of growing up. It's the time when your body changes from a child to an adult. For girls, it takes about five years to get all the way through puberty, but the most noticeable changes happen over about three years. Most girls start puberty between the ages of eight and twelve. Most boys start between nine and fourteen. So remember, sometimes it may seem like you are the only one dealing with body changes, but *everyone* goes through puberty.

It's no secret that the reason your child body has to change into an adult body is so that one day you will be able to have babies if you want to. It takes a lot of time for the body to change and prepare itself to make a baby. That's why all these changes start when you are young. Puberty allows your body to grow and develop so it will be prepared to grow a new life when you are older and ready to start a family.

How Does Puberty Start? (Ready ... Set ... Go!)

Puberty actually starts in the brain, but you can't see or feel the very beginning. It all begins when the brain sends out *chemical messengers* to the rest of your body. These messengers are called hormones, and they start all the changes. There are hormones that tell your body to grow faster, hormones that tell your breasts to start growing, hormones that tell hair to sprout in new places, and hormones that cause new smells to creep out of your armpits. There are other hormones working every day to make even more changes happen. Before you even notice the first change, your hormones have been working, slowly and steadily, for a couple of years!

When Will These Changes Happen?

We bet you're wondering exactly when the changes will start or stop. Unfortunately, there's no one answer that works for everyone. Just as you are unique in the things you like to do, the sound of your laugh, and what you like to eat for breakfast, your body is just as unique. That means it will follow its own schedule—yours and yours alone. And your best friend will have *her* own schedule. And the girl that sits next to you in math class will have her own schedule, too. Some of your friends may go through the changes when you do, but some will be way behind or way ahead of you. The cool thing is that everyone goes through the same stuff, but each girl has her own unique schedule and her own unique body when puberty is over.

Just to remind you how one-of-a-kind you are and how different even your best friends may be, fill out the Think About It chart below.

Think About It

	Me	Friend 1	Friend 2	Friend 3
Eye color				
Favorite singer or band				
Favorite breakfast food				
Hobbies				
Favorite animal				
Fears				
Favorite vacation spot				
Best school subject				
Favorite game				
Favorite teacher				

Looking over the chart, you'll probably notice you have a lot in common with your buddies—some of these things might even be part of the reason you are such good friends. But you probably also have some differences. Do the differences make you not like them anymore? Of course not! It's just part of the stuff that makes each of you interesting. If we were all exactly the same, things would get way boring.

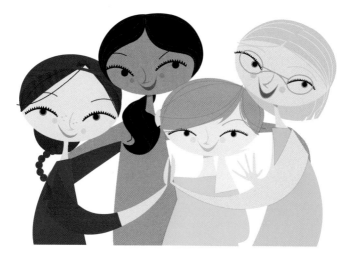

How are you and your friends different yet the same? Maybe you are quiet, and your best friend is a total crack up, but you both love to dance. Or maybe you have a natural talent for math, and she is a great artist, but you both play soccer. Just as good friends have similarities and differences in their looks and their personalities, you'll realize that *all* the girls around you have similarities and differences as they go through puberty.

You have to remember that being different is normal, even when it doesn't always feel that way. And it's really neat the way we all go through the same changes, but on our own schedule and with different results that make each of us unique.

You have to remember that being different is normal, even when it doesn't always feel that way.

Do Your Feet Hurt?!

YOU WILL KNOW PUBERTY HAS STARTED when your feet hurt. Does puberty *make* your feet hurt? No, but tight shoes do. And guess what the very first noticeable sign of puberty is for most girls? Their feet start growing! Those hormones that tell your body to grow faster make your hands and feet grow first. So when you find yourself outgrowing your sneakers faster than normal, you can smile to yourself and know puberty's starting! We'll talk more about how you'll grow in Chapter 3.

What's My Brain Got to Do with Puberty??

Remember how it all started in your brain? Well, as your brain starts sending out the messenger hormones, it starts going through some changes of its own. That means your brain is actually growing smarter and getting ready to learn totally new

things. Cool! Starting around
age eleven, most girls' and boys'
brains are able to understand
things that didn't make sense
when they were younger. You
can start to understand things
you can't necessarily see, like "fairness" and
"beliefs."

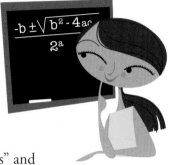

Your brain also begins to understand more complicated things like algebra. Ask your teachers! They know that it's pretty impossible to teach even simple algebra to a first grader, but by middle school, most kids "get it."

All these brain changes also mean that you are able to think about things that happened in the past and learn from them. Then you can take what you learned and use it to help you make new decisions.

For example, let's say your parents asked you to clean your room before you went to spend the night at a friend's house. In the excitement of packing for the sleepover, you forgot to clean your room and raced out of the house when your friend's mom came to pick you up. The next day, your mom was pretty angry and made you wait a month before you could have another sleepover. By the end of that month, when your mom asked you to clean your room, you remembered what happened last time. You quickly got to work cleaning so you wouldn't miss any more fun sleeping over with your friends. Instead of forgetting about the punishment and doing the same old things over and over, your brain clicked in and said, "Hold on! Remember what happened last time?! If you let that happen again, you'll miss all the fun!"

And making good decisions is what helps you stay smart and safe.

When you were six, that conversation in your head probably wouldn't have happened. Now that you are starting to think in a more mature way, you are able to make better decisions. And making good decisions is what helps you stay smart and safe. For now, this part about thinking better may sound a little confusing, but as your brain grows in puberty, it will make more sense.

Moods and Me

Besides being your body's "computer," your brain is also the place where most of your emotions come from. All the growth and change in your brain will also make your emotions change a lot. Emotions describe the way you feel, like being happy, sad, angry, embarrassed, or scared. Everyone experiences a lot of different emotions over time—and even within one day. In puberty, you may find that you experience new emotions and that they

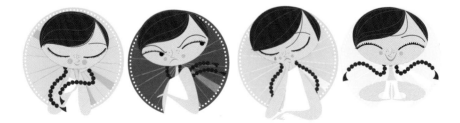

may feel stronger than they've ever been. They can also change more quickly. They can even seem really confusing.

If you find yourself laughing and having fun one minute, then crying or really angry the next, it doesn't mean you're crazy! It's probably more related to your emotions growing just like the rest of your body.

Around puberty, it's normal to have mixed up and changing feelings. What's most important is that you see the emotion as a reaction to something you've experienced. You also need to learn to "let your emotions out" in a safe and healthy way. We talk about that more below. Some people blame bad or changing moods on "hormones," but at your age, it's really just because of the growing going on in your noggin. And like most of those other changes happening around puberty, being "moody" is pretty normal.

Feelings

Besides being moody during puberty, you will have lots of different feelings throughout the day. You may feel happy, sad, embarrassed, angry, nervous, or even jealous. Feelings, even negative ones like jealousy, are normal. What matters most is the way you express your feelings.

What matters most is the way you express your feelings.

When you are happy, you may smile, laugh, high-five, or dance. The "happy" feelings are easy to express and people like seeing you express them. The "bad" feelings, like being sad, disappointed, or angry, are just as important to express, but it's hard to express them and not hurt other people.

What do you do when you are angry? It's easy to express your anger in unhealthy ways, like yelling, screaming, hitting, gossiping, and being mean to people who had nothing to do with the reason you're angry. But there are also healthy ways to express your anger, like taking some deep breaths to calm down, writing in your journal, or even going for a run to clear your head. If you really feel like yelling and screaming, go ahead and yell into your pillow or go outside and yell, but don't yell or scream at another person. It never helps anything. Once you have calmed down a bit, it might help to write down the reason you got angry and some solutions that can prevent it from happening again. If your anger involves a friend, you may need to explain it to her after you've calmed down.

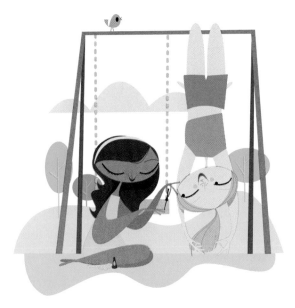

Feeling Girly?

Along with your emotions, the way you feel about yourself may be changing, too. Some girls like the body changes taking place and some don't. Some girls want to act more grown-up and some don't. How do you feel about your own growth and changes?

A common feeling for girls going through puberty is to feel more "girly." That means you might become more interested in the way you look. You may become more interested in changing your hairstyle, painting your nails, or dressing differently. Other times, you might want to put on a baseball hat, play soccer, or climb a tree instead. If you sometimes want to act more "girly" or grown-up, but other times just want to be more like a little kid, that's perfectly normal, too.

There are some girls who never want to wear makeup or paint their nails. Are they weird? Nope. They're just as normal as anyone else. As we said before, all these changes will happen but everyone reacts to the changes in their own unique way. There is no right way or wrong way to feel or act because you're a girl; there are just different ways.

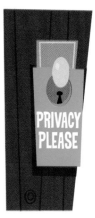

Feeling Weird?

Since puberty is a time of so many changes, it is perfectly natural to feel a little weird or worried about all that's going on. You might feel more modest. That means you want privacy when you dress and undress. Sometimes, you might even feel embarrassed about your changing body parts. It's also normal to be curious about how your friends' bodies are changing and whether your changes are like theirs. The most important thing to remember is that all the changes happen a little differently for everyone. So if your changes are not exactly like your friends', don't worry. Most girls feel at least a little worried or weird at some point during this whole puberty thing. Just remember, your body is doing exactly what it is meant to do on its own schedule. If you see it as something positive (which it really is), you'll get through puberty feeling happier and more excited about all the amazing things that your body is doing—just as it was meant to.

CHAPTER 2

Can We Be Friends?

Riley

IT IS SATURDAY. It is sunny and I am headed to the park. Life is good!

CJ and John are already there. "Hey, Riley, come on. Let's go," they call to me. I park my bike at the rack and hurry over to them.

"Hey guys. What's up?" I ask

"Nothing." They reply in unison.

We silently make our way to the field.

We separate to form a triangle. CJ throws the Frisbee to John who in turn throws it to me. We do this for a while then head over to the basketball court looking for a pick-up game. We find one in no time. CJ and John are great at steals and rebounding. They always pass to me. I'm the shooter. I fire a long three-pointer in. Swish—nothing but net!

One of our opponents starts teasing his teammate.

"You are getting schooled by a girl!"

The kid replies, "Riley's not really a girl. She doesn't count."

We finish playing. I keep thinking about his words.

When I get home, I head to my room and take off my baseball hat. I pull my hair out of the ponytail and look at myself in the mirror. I *am* a girl. I wish people would remember that. I never used to care what other people thought. Lately, though, their comments are starting to bother me. I love sports and hanging out with the guys, but I still want people to think of me as a girl. Maybe I need to start hanging around other girls more. I decide that is exactly what I will do.

Monday morning, I wake up early and take a really long time getting ready. I blow-dry my long, light brown hair. From the back of my closet, I pull out the shirt my Aunt Sue gave me. Never thought that I would be caught dead in something so girlie girlish, but it does look way better on. No ponytail and T-shirt for me today.

At lunch, I walk right past CJ and John's table. I sit down with several girls. The girls look at me like I am a visiting alien, but allow me to sit without a protest. They talk to me very politely with syrupy sweet smiles on their faces. The discussion is all about which character is hotter—the vampire or the werewolf. I am a little lost. I haven't read the book, but I try to act interested. They talk so much, they barely touch their food. Definitely not like the boys!

Later I am in the bathroom, in one of the stalls. Tess and Beth, two of the girls from lunch, come in.

"Did you see Riley in that outfit? Who does she think she is?"

"I know. Like, really."

"And does she think she can just sit with us?"

"I know."

"She doesn't even have the first clue about anything."

"Like really."

I freeze. They are talking about *me*! I can't believe it. They were nice to my face and then they talk about me behind my back. Girls are so weird. Girls are so mean. I don't know what to do. I stay in the stall until they are gone. I will not cry. I will not let them know that they hurt me. But they did.

⁓

Who do you eat lunch with? Who do you play with at recess? Who do you like having sleepovers with? Is there someone new you'd like to invite to your birthday party this year? As you get older, it's fun to make new friends and get to know more people.

Most likely, you will have some good friends and you will have some not so good friends. And even you, yourself, will be a really good friend sometimes, and not such a good friend other times. Nobody can be perfect all the time, but learning to be a good friend takes time and practice.

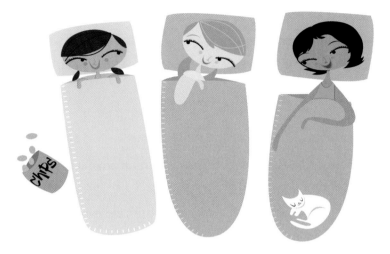

In this chapter, we'll talk about good friends and bad friends and how to deal with both. We want *you* to learn to be a good friend and be true to yourself, and to avoid being a negative or bad friend. You don't have to please everyone or be everyone's best friend, but there's no reason to be mean or ugly to other people. That doesn't do any good for anyone!

Bullies

You've probably heard about bullies. Most people think of a bully as someone who picks on other people or starts a fight—a big kid with anger problems and a mean streak. But that's not the usual type of bully lurking in the halls of your school. More likely, a bully can look just like you and even have a lot of "friends." In the story that started this chapter, did you see Tess and Beth as bullies? If Riley was nice to the girls at lunch, why do you think Tess and Beth were talking about her later?

So, what makes someone a bully? It's complicated. Even the nicest, prettiest, smallest girl can act like a bully sometimes. All it takes is doing or saying something that makes another person feel bad about herself. It may be on purpose, but it can also happen by accident.

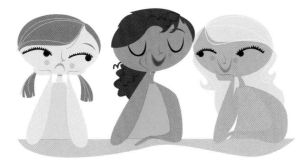

Unfortunately, there will always be people in this world who aren't so nice. And sometimes, even nice people may do something that seems mean. A lot of times, a girl or boy can act mean to someone, but later realize that they feel bad about the way they acted. A good friend will apologize for being mean or unfair. It's all part of learning how to act. Being a good friend takes some work. As friendships are changing, it's important to do your best to avoid being a "mean girl" or bully.

If bullying doesn't have to involve starting a fight, what exactly is it? All of the things below are considered bullying:

* Telling a story about someone that isn't true
* Saying mean things about someone to their face or behind their back

Being a good friend takes some work.

* Being in a group that doesn't allow others to join in

* Hurting someone's feelings on purpose

* Whispering or telling secrets in front of others who don't know what you're saying

What are some other ways that you have seen bullying happen?

Why Bully?

There are a million different ways that girls and boys can be mean to each other. Why on earth do they want to do that?

Most of the time, the mean girl or bully acts the way they do for different reasons.

* She may be jealous of something you have or can do, so she makes fun of it. That makes it seem less "great" to her. Then she feels better about not having whatever it is.

* She may feel badly about herself and thinks she will feel better by making you feel badly about yourself.

* She may be copying the way she has been treated by others.

* She may believe she is powerless, and hurting someone else makes her feel powerful.

* She may think she is being funny.

Whatever the reason for bullying, it's never funny. It's just plain wrong to hurt someone's feelings on purpose. It doesn't feel good for the person being bullied. And the bully may even realize that it doesn't make her feel better about herself either. It can't.

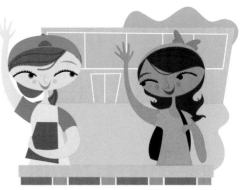

Nothing feels better than making someone feel great! Make their day! Watch them smile. Laugh with them. Include them in your fun. There's no better way to feel great than to be a good friend to others. By setting a good example, you will encourage your friends to do the same. It's good for everyone.

> There's no better way to feel great than to be a good friend to others.

Cliques: Good or Bad?

Friends tend to hang out together. That's part of friendship. But if you always hang out with the same group of friends, the group may be considered a clique. Cliques can be good or bad. Good groups tend to welcome new friends and work together to do good things. It's easy to see that a group can do more than one person can when it comes to things like projects or helping others. Groups are also fun because there's a lot of variety and more fun to go around.

Then why does the word "clique" seem so negative? When does a group of friends become a problem? The biggest problem

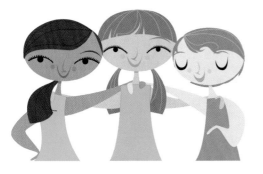

with cliques is that the group becomes so "tight" that they don't let others join in on their fun. This is called *exclusion,* and it hurts the ones being left out. Remember, exclusion is a type of bullying.

Do you only let certain girls sit at your lunch table or hang out with you at recess? What if someone not in your group tries to join in? Do you have friends who ignore her or even get up and walk away?

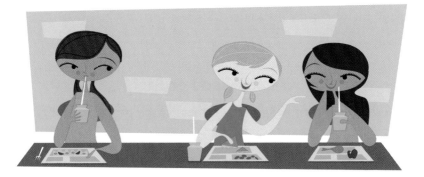

If you've ever been in a situation like this, you've seen how exclusion works. There is a girl who is being excluded. There are "bullies" who exclude her. And there are "bystanders" who watch this happen but don't really do anything bad OR good. Even as a bystander it can feel bad and it's hard to know how to stand up for the one being left out.

Being in a Clique Is Complicated

If you have ever stood by and watched another girl's feelings get hurt by your friends—and wanted to help her but didn't—then you know that being a bystander is complicated. If you decide to help out the excluded girl, your friends may exclude *you* for not sticking by them. If you don't help the girl, you feel badly for her. You might even feel guilty for not helping. It's normal to have mixed feelings in a situation like this.

How can you keep your friends but still do what feels right? First of all, friends who exclude others are not the best friends to have. One choice is to find another group that isn't so exclusive. Leaving a "mean" group and finding a better group for you may be really hard, but also really rewarding. What usually happens is that you find the best friends ever in a group of girls who like including others and enjoy different types of friends.

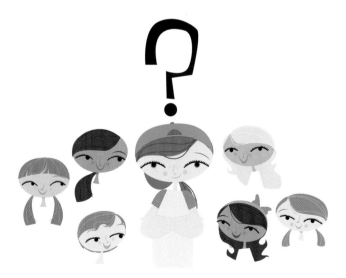

On the other hand, you might be able to help your friends see that it is mean to exclude others. Sometimes girls don't even realize that their group is being exclusive or mean. Saying something like, "How would you feel being left out?" can make them more understanding and change the way they act. That is a great thing for everyone involved!

What if the "leader" of the group gets mad at you and threatens to never talk to you again or do something even worse? It's a perfect time to lose her as a friend. You need to stand up for yourself and speak up against the bully. You need to find your "voice," even though it can be scary. If you feel scared or don't know how to get a bully to leave you or someone else alone, talk with a teacher, parent, or other adult that you trust.

Whether you are being bullied or are just a bystander, speaking up takes courage. If you're being bullied, you might just stand there, you might cry, or maybe you might run away. It's hard to speak up for yourself sometimes. Having courage can take time and practice. Practice? Yep. It can really help to think about some comebacks to use if you're bullied or if you're a bystander. See some of our suggestions in "Finding Your Anti-Bully Voice."

Having courage can take time and practice.

Finding Your Anti-Bully Voice

What to Say to a Bully

✳ "Why don't you grow up?"

✳ "Do you like being a bully?" or "Do you like being mean?"

✳ "I'm sorry, you seem to be having a bad day."

✳ Say nothing, show no reaction, and just walk away like it had no effect on you.

What to Say if You're a Bystander

✳ "I can't believe you said that!"

✳ "How would you feel if someone did that to you?"

✳ Just say the bully's name in a way that shows you disagree or are surprised at what she's saying, like, "Tess!?!?!?"

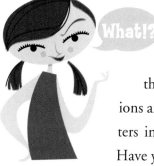

Being a Good Friend

Being good friends doesn't mean you always have to agree on everything and like the same things. Even the best of friends can have different opinions and different likes and dislikes. What matters in friendships is treating each other well. Have you heard of the golden rule? Treat others

Treat others the way you would like to be treated.

the way you would like to be treated. It doesn't mean treat others the way they treat you. So you can go first. Think about these "good friend" practices:

* If you treat others nicely by being helpful and friendly, they will more likely be helpful and friendly to you.

* If you know you hurt your friend's feelings, then be sure to say you are sorry. You would want to be treated the same way if your feelings were hurt.

* If there's a new girl in your class, be one of the first to be her friend. You would appreciate someone being your friend if you were new.

Remember, if you treat others in mean ways, you'll get it right back. By living the golden rule, however, you can be a great example for others of what a true friend is.

Finding Good Friends

Don't expect everyone to be your BFF, and don't feel like you have to be everyone's best friend. It takes time to grow great friends. Having even one great friend is better than having a lot of so-so friends.

It's also just fine to have friends that are boys, but not "boy-friends." Lots of girls are buddies with boys. Their friendships may be based on liking the same things, being neighbors, having

similar hobbies, or playing the
same sport. Sometimes girls
who have friends that are
boys are teased about
having a "boy friend."
Friends are friends, and
the teasers need to grow
up. You can tell them we said
so!

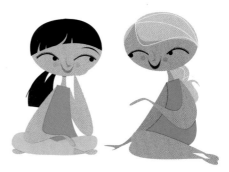

By being a good friend, you will find good
friends. Good friends bring out the best in you.
They are the girls and boys you can talk with and
trust. They are honest and stand up for you. They

Good friends bring out the best in you.

don't talk behind your back. They are happy when things go well
for you. They think your weird habits, your goofy laugh, and
your crazy hair are just fine. Good friends are the ones who know
and like the true you.

CHAPTER 3

Body Talk

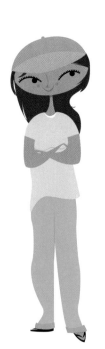

Brianna

"BRIANNA, HONEY, TIME TO WAKE UP."

"Argh," I moan and then roll over.

"Come on, Sweetie. You need to get ready for school."

"I'm up," I say, and my mom leaves the room. Oh man, am I tired! Morning comes too fast. I pull the pillow over my head and grant myself five more minutes of sleep.

"Brianna!" my mom yells. "What are you doing?"

"What? Oh, sorry Mom. I'm getting up now."

I quickly take a shower and get dressed. Today I am wearing one of my brother's T-shirts. It is way too big for me, just the way I like it! I grab a piece of toast and my mom drives me to school. As she glances over at me, I know before she speaks that she disapproves of my outfit. I let out a little sigh and brace myself for her lecture. Surprisingly, she doesn't say a word. My mom doesn't like me to wear these baggy clothes. She is always saying that I have such a beautiful figure, I shouldn't cover it up. Well, she doesn't know what it is like to be the only one in the grade with a "figure." I hate being so tall and grown-up looking.

At school, I stop by my locker. Claire and Lily are there. They both give me friendly smiles and say hello. I smile back, but I don't feel like it. I wish I were more like them. Claire is really cute and petite. I feel like an Amazon woman next to her. Lily always looks so pulled together and perfect. Next to Lily, I feel way frumpy.

The social studies class is going on a field trip. Our teacher Mrs. Cox has a stack of T-shirts with the school logo on them. She wants us all to wear them. My stomach starts fluttering. What size shirt does she have for me? Oh, I so do not want to be here. Mrs. Cox hands out all of the shirts, and then sends us off in groups of four to the bathroom to change. When it is my turn, I take my shirt and dash ahead. My shirt fits, and that is the problem. I think about my options. It is way too hot to wear a sweatshirt. I hate the thought of people staring at me. I take a deep breath and tell myself that maybe I'm making too big a deal of this whole thing.

As I walk back into class, I feel eyes staring at me. Or am I imagining it? I slump back down in my seat.

"Hey Brianna—nice rack!" Andrew whispers to me.

Ahhh. What does that mean? Oh no. Please tell me this isn't happening. Is he talking about my chest? I ignore him. I keep my arms folded over my body for the rest of the day. Somehow I make it through and my torture day is finally over.

Later, we are sitting at the table for dinner. Mom, Dad, my big brother, David, and me. My mom likes us to go around the table telling our good news of the day. As if I have any good news to share today! When it is my turn, I ask if I can be excused.

"Brianna, you haven't even finished your dinner yet. What's the matter?"

"Nothing," I mumble.

My mom looks at me. She knows something's up. She always does. Finally, I can't take it anymore.

"Can I be excused? Please?" I am begging now.

"May I be excused," she corrects me. I am about to crumble, but she adds, "All right, you *may* be excused."

David quickly adds, "Me, too. Can, I mean, may I be excused, too?"

"Okay, okay, but clear your plates."

We take off before she can change her mind.

Once we are upstairs, I turn to David and blurt, "Andrew said that I had a nice rack. What does that mean?"

David tries to suppress a chuckle. I glare at him.

"What? I didn't say anything," he says. "But that's just the way guys talk. It means you have a nice . . . um . . . chest." David cups both hands over his own chest as he speaks.

My eyes fill with water. I am beyond embarrassed that Andrew really was talking about that.

"Hey, hey. Brie, don't be upset. The guy is a total idiot to say that to you."

All guys are idiots, I think to myself.

"And if Andrew or any other big mouth ever says anything rude to my little sister again, I'll shut him up myself!" David is practically screaming now. It makes me feel good that he would stand up for me.

"Thanks, David," I say as some of the tears spill out.

He gives me a couple of quick pats on the back, like I'm one of his teammates. Then he offers me one of the dirty shirts on his floor to dry my eyes. For some reason we both think that is the funniest thing. Now I am laughing and crying! Maybe all boys are not idiots; my brother is pretty cool!

Since there are a lot of changes going on with your body, you'll want to make sure you know the scoop on all your parts—and all the nicknames that you might hear about them (like "rack"). You probably already know most of the names for the parts of your body. You learned most of them when you were a toddler, right? Remember the song, "Head, shoulders, knees and toes, knees and toes?" You're singing it now, aren't you? It's so cute when a little baby can point and name

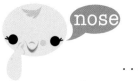 their parts, but what about the parts that people don't usually talk about. You know . . . those personal, private, covered-up parts.

Yep, those.

Can you name all the parts *down there*? Or do you just point or call the whole area some silly "nickname"? We've probably heard most of the silly names there are for a girl's "private" parts: Coochie. Front Fanny. Booboo. Girly Gadgets. Pee Pee. Tee Tee. Pocketbook. Wahoo, Hooha, and Hoo hoo. What names have you heard?

Okay, okay! When you stop laughing, read on.

Why do we get all embarrassed or silly when we have to talk about our parts *down there*? A lot of times, people get embarrassed because they don't know the real names. Sometimes, it just seems embarrassing to talk about parts that we're not supposed to show.

Remember, everything that your bathing suit covers is considered "private." Those parts are covered because they are not for anyone to see or touch, except you. But even those private parts have names, and it's important for you to know them. That way, if you're having a problem or a question about your changing body, you'll know how to talk with your parent or your nurse or doctor if you need help or answers.

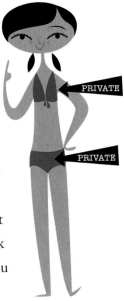

Besides silly nicknames, there are also some not-so-nice words that some people use to describe private body parts or things that those parts do. You'll hear some kids or adults use those words from time to time. Some kids think they sound "cool" or older when they use words like that. Some just don't have any respect for our amazing bodies and use disrespectful words.

For girls who are in-the-know, like you, there's no need to use "naughty" words at all! In fact, using "bad" or "dirty" words to describe your body parts just makes those parts seem dirty or wrong. And guess what? There's nothing dirty or wrong about your girl parts. Just remember that they are there for very important reasons, and without them, you'd have some major problems!

Girl Parts: Up Top

Let's start at the top. When we talk about girl parts, most people think of the "down there" parts. But we have special parts up top, too. And like other body parts, they also have some nicknames, like boobs, bosoms, and plenty of other silly and even disrespectful names. But we prefer to call them breasts.

First of all, each of your breasts has a couple of parts of its own. On each breast, there is a circle of darker skin with a bump in the middle. The bump is called the nipple, and the darker skin around each nipple

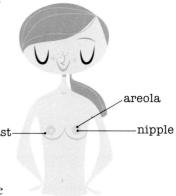

is called the areola (uh REE oh luh). It kind of looks like a target. Maybe that's to help a new baby find it since the main reason our breasts grow is to prepare our body to make breast milk if we have a baby.

Breast milk is definitely the best food there is for a newborn baby. Whether a woman decides to feed her baby breast milk or baby formula depends on a lot of things, sometimes just a choice she makes. The great news is that all breasts, whether big or small, can make breast milk. That's the real reason they are there.

Girl Parts: "Down There"

Now let's move to the "down there" parts. When it comes to seeing your own private parts, we have to admit that boys have it easier. As you can imagine, on a boy, his private parts are dangling right there in front. He can see them. He even has to hold his penis to aim into the toilet (hopefully!) when he urinates (that's the medical word for pee). So, for a boy, his parts are pretty easy to see and touch.

Girls are different (duh!). Our parts are kind of hidden around a corner between our legs. They're not easy to see, and we really haven't had to learn to hold them, watch them, or aim them anywhere. So for girls, those parts may seem a bit mysterious. Well, there's no need to keep it a mystery. They are *your* parts, right? Nothing about your own body needs to be a mystery!

Those "Down There" Parts Have Real Names

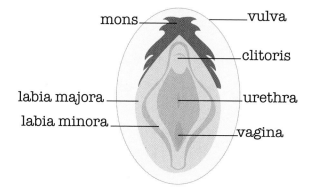

The first thing to learn is that there is one name for the "group" of girl parts down there (just like your face includes your eyes, nose, mouth, chin, cheeks, eyebrows, and other things). The whole area between your legs that makes up your girl parts is called the *vulva* (**VUHL** vuh). Just like your face has all those smaller parts, the vulva includes a lot of different parts, too.

If you look down to try to see what's there, the main thing you can see is a fatty bump called the *mons* (monz). It's fatty and soft to protect the bone that is underneath. If you push on it, you can feel the bone it covers. It's also the place where your pubic hair will grow (if it hasn't already) into the shape of a triangle (more about hair in Chapter 5).

Below the mons between your legs, you can see the beginning of two flaps or folds that meet in the middle. They are closed but can be spread open, kind of like lips. And guess what they are called? Our large lips. Well, sort of! In Spanish, the word for lip is *labia* and the word for big is *majora*. And the real name for those flaps or folds is labia majora (LAY be uh Ma JOR ah). They are the "big lips" that cover some other sensitive parts that are beneath and between them.

Now, if the labia majora are spread apart, there are some smaller folds of skin in there. They are called the labia minora (LAY be uh Mi NOR ah). I bet you can figure out what that means. *Labia* means lip. *Minora* means minor or small. You got it! They're the smaller lips that also help protect some other sensitive parts.

At the top of the labia minora is a bump called the clitoris (CLIT or us). The clitoris holds many nerves that make it feel tingly or tickly when it's touched. Sometimes you see baby girls touching that area because it feels good to them. The clitoris is the part of the vulva that is most sensitive to touch.

Between the labia minora are two holes. The hole closest to the front is where your urine (pee) comes out. It's called the urethra (your REE thra), and it can be pretty sensitive to touch or chemicals. If it gets touched or hit, it hurts! The pink skin around it is also really sensitive and can burn if soaps or other chemicals get in it. If you ever have a lot of stinging or burning around the urethra when you urinate, you need to let your parent know so you can see a doctor. Burning when you urinate can sometimes mean you have an infection.

The hole below the urethra is the vagina (va JI nuh). It's the opening where a baby comes out, and it's also the part that connects the outside girl-parts to the inside girl-parts. The open-ing can have a lot of different looks, but usually it's just a small hole. Some girls may have a vaginal opening that looks more like several small holes or maybe two holes side by side. The opening might be a hole in the middle or a little off to one side. All of these variations are normal, but just another individual differ-ence between people.

We know you're probably wondering, "A whole baby can fit through that little hole that is the vagina?" We know it doesn't seem possible, but when a woman is pregnant and starts to have her baby, the vagina can stretch and stretch to be big enough to let a baby out. It's one more amazing thing about our bodies!

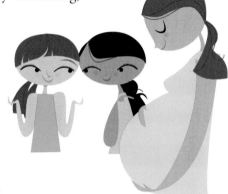

There is one other way that babies can come out, but it's not the "natural" way. It's a type of surgery called a cesarean section (also called a c-section), and it means that a doctor cuts an open-ing in the lower part of the mother's belly to take the baby out. There are different reasons why some women need a c-section, but most babies are born through the vagina. Now, that's some-thing amazing!

Uranus

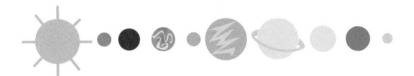

THERE IS ONE MORE HOLE "down there," but it's not considered part of the vulva, because both boys and girls have one. That's the hole we have a bowel movement (poop) through. It's called the anus. You may notice that some kids giggle when the science teacher talks about the planets and mentions "Uranus." Your science teacher may even giggle. Something about that just makes us laugh sometimes. It's okay. We just want to make sure you know the correct words for *all* your parts.

Check Out Your Body!

Now that you know all the parts that should be *down there*, you might want to look for yourself. It's normal to be curious. Sometimes you can settle your curiosity by taking a look. That way, you can make sure all your parts are present.

So how on earth do you do that? The only way we know is to get a mirror. Find a private place with good lighting, or you may want to use a flashlight. It's definitely something to do alone because you're looking at those *private* parts. It might feel weird, but it is your body, right? You need to know what it looks like, and you'll feel better knowing you have all the parts that you just learned about.

We bet you'll find all the parts that are supposed to be there, but if you have any questions or worries, you might want to ask your mom or your doctor. Being able to go to an adult you trust with your questions and worries is really important. This is not something that your friends will know any better than you.

There's Even More "Inside"!

Wait! There's even more! You know how we named all the outside body parts? What about what's on the inside? Like your heart, lungs, brain, bones? Even though you can't see any of those parts, you know they are in there and working, right? And, yep, you guessed it: there are girl-parts on the inside, too. Like your brain or lungs, you can't see the inside girl-parts, but they're in there and ready to work. As you go through puberty, you'll even start to *know* they're working by the new things that start going on with your body.

There are lots of long names for some of the inside parts, but they all work together to allow us to have babies one day. The main parts are the uterus, where a baby grows, and the ovaries, where the eggs that are necessary for a baby are stored. Then

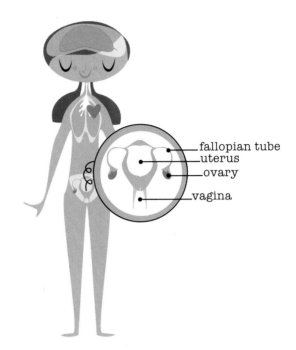

there are tubes and openings that connect everything together so the baby on the inside can get to the outside through the vagina. Here's a picture of how they all fit together.

You Are Amazingly Strong!

Now you know we're as wonderfully complicated on the inside as we are on the outside. And you know what else? These inside parts are amazing. Think about it. The uterus is the place where a baby grows. And remember, the baby eventually comes out of the vagina, which you may have noticed by now is a pretty small opening. How in the world can a seven- or eight-pound baby get out of there? It takes great muscle strength, and your body is becoming stronger than you could ever imagine.

To grow a baby and help it get out of the body, it takes a uterus. The uterus is made of amazingly strong and coordinated muscles. Right now, your uterus is about the size of your fist. Not so big, right? But when a woman is pregnant, the baby growing in her uterus causes it to stretch bigger and bigger. Have you ever seen a pregnant woman and noticed how big her belly is? Sometimes it looks as big as a basketball, or even bigger! All that bigness comes from the growing baby inside her uterus.

It takes great muscle strength, and your body is becoming stronger than you could ever imagine.

After the baby has finished developing and growing (which takes about nine or ten months!), it's time for the baby to be born. To make that happen, the muscles in the uterus start to squeeze. The uterus squeezes every few minutes, harder and harder, until it finally helps push the baby out of the vagina. Pretty incredible!

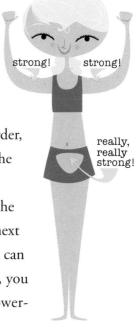

strong!   strong!

really,
really
strong!

That means the uterus is probably one of the strongest muscles in the human body. So, next time a boy thinks he's stronger than you, you can just smile to yourself and know that, as a girl, you have a muscle that is stronger and more powerful than he could ever even think about being! Now that's real girl power!

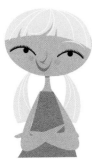

You Are Incredible!

So you see, your body has a lot of parts, and though it may seem a bit complicated, what a miraculous body it is! You are made so incredibly well, and your body can do special and amazing things! You may not always feel so great about your body parts, especially as they change. But when you look at all your parts and how they work together to make us girls do the cool and extraordinary things that girls do . . . you'll just have to smile from your head, to your shoulders, to your knees and toes!

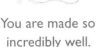

You are made so incredibly well.

CHAPTER 4

Bras!

Lily

"MOM, HAVE YOU SEEN MY CAMISOLE? I can't find it anywhere."

"It's in the wash."

"What? Oh no, what am I going to do?"

My mom walks into my room and sits on the foot of my bed.

"Lily, I know that you like to wear the camisole, but it really is time that we bought a bra for you."

"A bra?"

"Yes dear, a bra."

"But I don't want to wear a bra. The camisole is fine. Will it be clean in time for school?"

"I'll make a deal with you. I'll have your camisole ready, if you'll agree to go shopping for a bra with me after school tomorrow."

"That is blackmail."

"No, that is desperation!" Mom laughs as she walks out of the room.

I finish laying out my outfit for school tomorrow. Then I brush my teeth and climb into bed and . . .

. . . *White bras, pink bras, black bras. Lacy bras, satin bras, cotton bras. BRAS, BRAS, BRAS! There are hundreds of them. I am being attacked by bras. People are flinging them at me from every angle. I am covered in a mountain of bras. I try to dig my way out, but I cannot escape. I am gasping for air. HELP, I scream. I hear voices. They are calling my name and laughing. I recognize the voices—they are kids from school. They're all watching the bra attack. And they are not even helping. They are just laughing. . . .*

My alarm goes off. I wake up panting and out of breath. Thank goodness, it was just a dream! That was the strangest dream I've ever had.

My mom comes in my room carrying my clean camisole. "Here you are, honey. Now, remember our deal."

"Mom, I can't go shopping with you. It is too embarrassing. What if we see someone I know? I just can't do it."

"Lily, there is no need to be embarrassed."

"Please Mom. I really don't want to go. I'll wear a bra, but I don't want to go shopping for one."

"All right. How about if I bring home some bras for you to try on? Would that be better?"

"Yes! That would be great! Thanks Mom. I knew that you'd understand. You're the best."

She smiles at me and turns to leave the room.

"Oh and Mom, don't bring too many, Okay?"

We're pretty sure you know where your breasts are and what is going to happen to them in puberty, but let's go over it anyway, just to be complete! Remember how we mentioned those hormonal messengers that your brain sends out to your body parts when puberty begins? The first messages usually go to your feet and hands, telling them to grow, right? Guess where the next messages are sent? For most girls, the next messages are sent to the breasts.

Budding

There's one hormonal messenger in particular that makes your breasts grow. It's called estrogen (ES tro jin). Estrogen does other things besides work on your breasts, but for most girls, the first visible sign of puberty is a breast bud, and the "budding" normally starts sometime between ages eight and twelve. If you haven't seen any breast buds by age twelve, you should see your doctor for a checkup. Sometimes a medical problem can delay puberty, but medical treatment can usually get you back on track.

As breasts grow, they actually start out as hard knots under the areola. Most of the time, one breast buds first, so being lopsided is normal. The other breast usually buds about four to six months later and catches up.

During all this early growing, it's also normal for your breasts, particularly the bud (including your areola and nipples), to be a little sore sometimes. You may not even notice any soreness unless your breast gets bumped. If you have soreness or tenderness, it will usually go away after a couple of months, but it might return from time to time as your breasts continue to grow.

How Your Breasts Grow

Believe it or not, there was a doctor a long time ago that decided to describe the different stages of breast growth. His name was Dr. Tanner, and the stages of breast growth were named the Tanner Stages. Now why on earth was that necessary? Well, it actually helps you and your doctor know that your breasts are growing like they should. Tanner Stages can also help predict when some of your other puberty changes will happen. We talk about this in Chapter 5.

Let's look at the Tanner Stages for breast development. You can find the one you are in right now.

* **Tanner Stage 1:** There is no breast growth at all. Nothing has started. Nada. Zero. Nothing. Flat as a board. This is the way girls' breasts look before they start puberty.

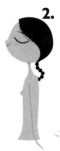

* **Tanner Stage 2:** This stage begins as soon as there is a breast bud. Sometimes you can feel the bud before you even see it. It may feel like a hard knot under the areola and nipple. And remember, it can be a little tender. Although one side usually buds at a time, both breasts should bud before you move into Stage 3.

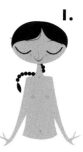

* **Tanner Stage 3:** After the breasts bud and the areola look larger and darker in color, there will be a small, fatty mound of breast tissue that forms on the chest and pushes the nipples and areola farther out. Sometimes the breasts look a little pointy, or sometimes they may look like a rounded mound.

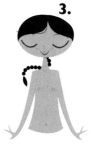

* **Tanner Stage 4:** This stage is sometimes hard to notice, but it's when the nipple and areola stick farther off the breast mound. It can look like there are two lumps making up each breast. Some girls never really notice this stage, and other girls think their breasts look weird in this stage.

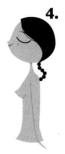

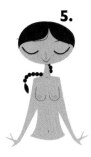

5.   ❋ **Tanner Stage 5:** This is the final stage when the breasts are grown and shaped like an adult woman's breasts. (And remember that there are all different sizes and shapes of breasts.) Once you reach this stage, your breasts may still have some growing to do. Most girls' breasts are not completely finished growing until they are seventeen or eighteen years old.

Big or Small?

A lot of girls worry about their breast size. Why should your breast size matter? If you worry about the size of your breasts, it's probably because you've seen or heard people comment about how big someone's breasts are. You may have noticed that a girl gets a lot of attention (good or bad) because of her breast size. Boys don't have breasts, so, of course, they're interested in them. Girls can say mean things sometimes about other girls' breasts. There may be teasing about someone who is flat chested or teasing about someone who has large breasts. Teasing about breasts is immature, but there will always be girls (and boys) who tease and bully. Besides teasing, sometimes people just go overboard and get silly about breasts.

The truth is, everyone's breasts are different: different shapes, different sizes. But all sizes of breasts can make breast milk for a newborn baby, and that's their real purpose, right? As your body changes and you develop breasts, you may feel like your breasts are too big or too small.

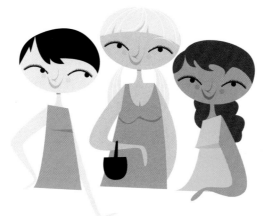

Often, girls with big breasts wish theirs were smaller. And girls with small breasts wish they had bigger ones. It's kind of like how girls with curly hair like straight hair, and girls with straight hair wish they had curls. Sometimes we just think that life would be better, easier, or more fun if we had something different. Guess what? Most of the time, that's just plain wrong.

We hear a lot of questions from girls about breasts. You might have some of the same questions. Here are some of those questions and our answers.

> Sometimes we just think that life would be better, easier, or more fun if we had something different.

If I develop breasts earlier than my friends, does that mean my breasts will be bigger than theirs when I'm grown? Not at all. Your breast size is mostly determined by your genetics (that means what you inherit through your mom and dad). Some girls that develop early may end up with smaller breasts, and some that develop later may have bigger ones. Besides genetics, your

breast size can also be affected by your weight. If you are overweight, you'll gain weight in your breasts as well as your tummy
and legs and everywhere else. If you are overweight and you lose
weight to become a healthier weight, you may find your bra size
decreases.

If my mom has small breasts, does that mean I will, too?
Maybe. Maybe not. Again, that depends on your genetics (there's
that word again). Even though your father doesn't have breasts,
you still inherit some of your size and shape from him and his
ancestors. So your breasts may be more like your aunts or grand-
mother on your dad's side, than like your mom's. Every person is
a new mixture of traits that makes each of us unique.

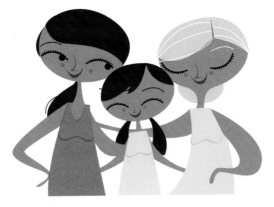

**Can I make my breasts grow more with pills or special
exercises?** No. The pills that are advertised to make breasts grow
actually have stuff in them that just make you gain weight. But
they can't just make you gain weight in your breasts. You'll gain
weight all over. Not a good idea! There also aren't any exercises

that make your breasts grow larger. Sometimes the muscles under the breasts may get bigger with a *lot* of exercise, but they don't change your breast size. Remember, it's not about how they look; it's about what they do!

When my breasts start to grow, does that mean I'll start my period soon? We haven't talked about periods yet (we'll get to that in Chapter 7), but the answer is no. When your breasts start to grow, that signals the beginning of puberty. It takes several years to get all the way through puberty. For most girls, periods start to happen about two to three years after you first notice breast buds.

Do I *have* to wear a bra? Once your breasts start to grow, it will be time to think about wearing a bra. Although you don't *have* to wear a bra, most girls feel more comfortable and more covered in one. Some girls are embarrassed about wearing a bra because they don't want anyone to know that they're developing. Remember that everyone develops, so you, your friends, and all the other girls around your age are in this together. It might feel a little embarrassing when it first starts, but before long, you'll get used to it!

When is it time to wear a bra? You might want to ask your mom, a big sister, or another adult you trust for advice. And see some of the answers we got from girls about when *they* decided it was time in "Time for a Bra!?" on the following page.

Time for a Bra!?

If you notice that your breasts are . . .

* ✳ beginning to show through your clothes
* ✳ starting to jiggle when you walk
* ✳ feeling heavy
* ✳ feeling sore

. . . it is probably time for you to go bra shopping!

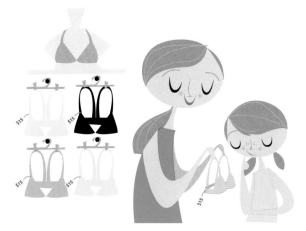

How do you feel about going shopping for a bra? Embarrassed, like Lily? Excited? Just another chore? Everyone has different feelings about it. If you don't want to look at bras in a store, maybe your mom or another adult you trust can bring some home for you to try on in the privacy of your own room. Leave the tags on and save the receipt so you can return the ones you don't like.

What Bra Type Are You?

Some girls like wearing tank tops with a built-in bra, or a cami (also called a camisole) instead of a real bra. Others like the security of a sports bra that prevents their breasts from wiggling or shaking. Some girls like to wear a bra with a little padding that helps keep their nipples from showing. Some like lacey bras, and some think lacey bras are too itchy. Some never want to wear a bra because it just seems too embarrassing. But for most girls, there comes a time when wearing a bra is more comfortable and less embarrassing than not wearing one.

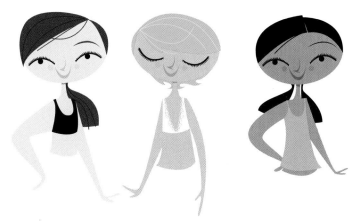

If you think you're ready for a bra, it's easy to start off with a stretchy camisole or sports bra. These will fit even the smallest breasts and still be comfortable. Once you have more breast tissue (Tanner Stages 3, 4, and 5), it will be important to buy the correct size.

Make sure your new bra holds all of your breast tissue in the "cups." A bra that is too small will be uncomfortable and will not provide good support for your growing breasts. Most girls get some "stretch marks" on their breasts or hips as they go through puberty, but a well-fitting bra can lessen the stretch marks that occur on your breasts.

> Most girls get some "stretch marks" on their breasts or hips as they go through puberty.

Bra sizes can be confusing and unpredictable. The best thing to do is to get fitted for one at a department or lingerie store. The ladies working there have been trained to measure and fit bras correctly, and they can help you find a bra that fits just right.

Bra sizes have two parts: a number and a letter. The number is a measurement of your rib cage around the part where the bottom of the bra fits. To get an idea of your size, you can use a tape measure and see how many inches around you are just under your breasts where the bra will sit. For young girls and teens, the sizes usually are anywhere from 32 to 38.

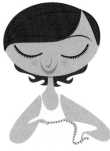

The letter part of the bra size tells how big the "cup" of the bra is. An A is the smallest cup size; then they get bigger as they go to B, C, D, and beyond. Since different brands of bras are made differently, you usually just have to try some on to find the right fit.

Like we said earlier, there are lots and lots of different types of bras out there. Check out "Your Bra Vocabulary" on the next page to learn about some of them.

Your Bra Vocabulary

Training bra. This bra doesn't really "train" anything, it just helps you get used to wearing one. A training bra is a small bra, usually with a cup size of A, AA, or AAA (small, smaller, smallest).

Natural bra. This natural or soft-cup bra is made of stretchy fabric without a padded or "formed" cup.

Jogging/Sports bra. This type of bra usually pulls over your head and is pretty snug. It keeps your breasts from bouncing around and hurting when you are running or very physically active. Some girls like to wear these all the time.

Underwire bra. This bra has a piece of hard plastic or wire under the cup. For girls with more breast tissue, the wire helps support the breasts and keep them from slipping below the cup.

Shelf bra. This is a "natural bra" that is built into a camisole or other clothing so you don't have bra straps showing under the spaghetti straps on the cami.

Padded bra. This bra has some padding built into it. Some girls wear these to help their clothes fit better or to make their breasts look a little larger. Some like them because they keep their nipples from showing.

Strapless bra. This is a bra without straps! Exactly like its name! This is the best type to wear if you have a strapless dress or top, or one with tiny straps.

Push-up bra. This bra pushes your breast tissue up and in to make them look fuller in the middle and create more of a "cleavage"—that's the line that forms between your breasts if they are large enough to meet in the middle. For example, the famous Wonder bra pushes breasts to the middle to create cleavage, but most women's breasts don't do that naturally. It takes padding, wires, and pushing from a special type of bra!

Demibra. This is a bra with a cup that covers mainly the bottom half of the breast only. Sometimes this smaller cup doesn't cover all of the areola.

Ze-bra. A black-and-white–striped bra. Just kidding!

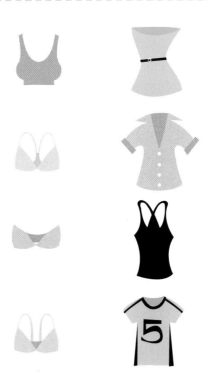

Now you know all about breasts and bras. And you should also know that there are all different shapes and sizes of breasts. The size and shape you have is just perfect for you, but your breasts might not be the same as your best friend's breasts. And it's a good thing we're not all exactly alike. Boring!

CHAPTER 5

"Down There"

Claire

I AM IN MY ROOM CHANGING. I hear the doorknob click. Then I hear knocking and banging on my door.

"Claire, what are you doing in there?" yells my mom. "Why is the door locked?"

"I'm getting dressed," I say. "I need some privacy."

"For heaven's sake, Claire. I'm your mother!"

"Mom, *please*," I plead.

"Claire, unlock this door, this instant!" She is shouting now.

I quickly scramble into my pj's and open the door. My mom is standing there with a funny look on her face. I thought that she was angry, but now she looks lost in thought.

"Guess my little girl is growing up," she says, as she kisses my forehead.

"Yea, guess so," I say with a shrug.

"Well, good night, Sweetie. Sleep tight." She waves and gently shuts the door as she leaves.

Huh? I'm not sure what that was all about. Moms can be so confusing!

I climb into my four-poster bed. I fluff up the pillows and wiggle my legs under the covers to get comfy. Then I reach over to the nightstand for my diary. I thumb through the pages until I find a clean one and begin writing.

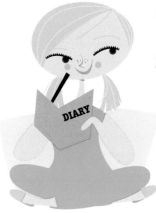

Dear Diary,

Today was a pretty good day. The rain finally stopped and we were able to go outside at recess. Brianna and I just sat on the swings and talked. Lily had to stay inside for a makeup test. I'm not supposed to tell another living soul this, Brianna made me promise, but I don't think you count (no offense). Brianna thinks that Michael Jamison is cute. She asked me if I thought he was cute, too. I'm not sure I really do (he's super tall and skinny), but I said that I did, not to hurt her feelings. She asked me who I liked and I said nobody. Guess that was two lies in a row. Just not ready to tell anyone about you-know-who yet.

I got an 88 on my math test. That was pretty good. Some people scored below 70. It was really hard. Think that I might be getting a little better at math. Still not my favorite subject.

Well, that's about it for news. I guess. There is something else that is way embarrassing. I really am not sure who to tell about it. Definitely not my mom. She would make a HUGE deal. It sort of is a big deal though. You know how I didn't think that I was ever going to show any signs that I was growing up or "developing"? I noticed one. I have a hair down there. You know, in my private place. It started off slowly. I thought it was a shadow. Now there are a lot more. Maybe I won't look like a seven-year-old forever. Maybe there's hope for me yet!

That's it for now.

Luv ya,

Claire

P.S. S.S.S. (sorry so sloppy)

Just like puberty signals the body to start growing breasts, it also causes some changes "down there" on the vulva and in the vagina. It's okay if you want to crinkle up your nose or say "ewwww," because this is all new stuff that does seem a little odd sometimes. But you have to remember that all these strange happenings are part of that very normal process called puberty!

New Stuff Down There

Have you noticed something new about you in your underwear? Don't panic. Around the time that your breasts start budding, you will start to notice some creamy white or yellow stuff in your underwear. It's coming from your vagina, and it's very normal! Just as the estrogen makes your breasts grow, it also works in the vagina to create this stuff that is called *vaginal discharge*. All girls and women have vaginal discharge. It might seem a little uncomfortable or embarrassing, because it can make you feel wet and sometimes a little sticky "down there."

Believe it or not, vaginal discharge is the way the vagina cleans itself. The discharge can change sometimes, too. It can be thin and watery; or clear, slimy, and mucousy (like the discharge from your nose!); or thick and creamy. Once it oozes out of the vagina (it's only a very little at a time), it can make your underwear wet, or it can dry up and be kind of crusty and yellow. It might have an odor, but it's not stinky.

Take Care Down There

For a lot of girls, vaginal discharge can be a little irritating to the sensitive skin on the vulva. Once there is hair on the mons and vulva, the hair helps pull the discharge away from your skin and makes it less irritating. If you have discharge, but not much hair, you may need to use a small pad, called a panty liner (see Chapter 8), to absorb the discharge. You can also put some diaper rash cream (or an over-the-counter ointment with zinc oxide) on the vulva to protect the skin from being bothered by the discharge.

If you notice a bad odor down there, it is usually from sweat or not washing well enough. The first remedy is always to wash well. When you wash your vulva, only use soap on the hairy area, but not inside the labia or around the vaginal opening. The tricky part is getting the dried discharge out from all those little folds. Use a soft washcloth and warm water, or sit in a tub and spread your labia apart to get the water in all those nooks and crannies.

Although bubble baths and scented body washes are nice sometimes, they can cause a lot of irritation to the sensitive skin around the vagina. If you take a bubble bath, just make sure to rinse the vulva off in fresh water (that means no bubbles or soap) before you get out of the tub.

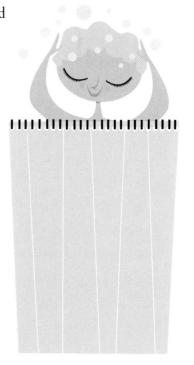

If you've washed well and still have problems with a bad odor, or if you have itching or burning around the vagina, you may need to see your doctor. These types of problems are usually easy to fix, so don't be afraid to get help.

Just remember that *all* girls going through puberty and *all* women have vaginal discharge. It's normal and just another part of growing up.

Hair Down There!

Remember the definition of puberty that meant "to grow hairy or mossy"? Yep, that's usually the next thing that happens once you start puberty. For some girls, especially those with dark hair or skin, the hair comes before the breast buds. You probably already know which parts become hairy, but you know us—we're gonna give you all the details!

As those hormone messengers are traveling around your body, they will cause you to start sprouting darker hairs on your mons and in your armpits. The hair on your mons is called *pubic* (PYOO bick) *hair*. You might also notice that the hairs on your legs are getting darker and thicker, too. (We'll talk more about armpit and leg hair in Chapter 6).

Dr. Tanner Again!

Remember Dr. Tanner? Well, he also came up with a way to "stage" the hair down there. We think that's a little weird, too, but it actually does help us understand how puberty progresses and when to expect other changes. Let's take a look at the stages, and you can see where you are.

✳ **Tanner Stage 1:** There is no hair other than a little "peach fuzz" that you've probably had all of your life. This is the way girls look before they enter puberty.

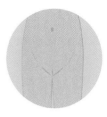

✳ **Tanner Stage 2:** There will be one, two, three . . . maybe up to five or six straight dark hairs. Definitely only a few, and you can count them (if you want to).

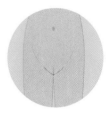

✳ **Tanner Stage 3:** There are more hairs and they start to get curly. There are usually more hairs than you would try to count, but you might be able to count them if you really really tried hard.

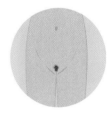

✳ **Tanner Stage 4:** There are way more hairs than you would ever be able to count, and the hairs grow in the shape of a triangle on the mons.

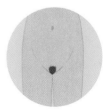

✳ **Tanner Stage 5:** This is the hair pattern that adult women have. The hair can spread up toward the belly button and down onto your thighs. It can also grow back toward your anus.

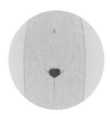

So there you have it. More than you ever wanted to know about your pubic hair. Everyone has it, but some people have more or less than others. If you have red hair, yours will be red. If you have blonde or brown hair, yours will be light or dark brown.

Need a Haircut?

There's really nothing to do about your pubic hair except keep it clean when you shower. At your age, there's no need to shave it, wax it, or remove it, unless you are already in Tanner Stage 4 or 5. Even then, it's still not necessary to do anything about it, but some girls are bothered by it. If it pokes out of your bathing suit or underwear, there are several ways to get rid of it, so you should talk with your mom about the best way for you.

If your pubic hair seems too long, you can trim it with some scissors. But be very careful. Remember how hard it is to see everything down there? Don't try to trim it too close, or you might accidentally cut your skin. Ouch! There's no reason to ever remove all of it since it helps protect the sensitive skin of your vulva.

This may seem like the most embarrassing stuff that happens in puberty. It's private. It's not something we chat about, and it's definitely different. Sometimes, though, you just need to know that all these changes are normal. Welcome to puberty!

CHAPTER 6

Squeaky Clean and Sparkling

Brianna

SUNSCREEN? CHECK!

Towel? Check!

iPod? Check!

All set.

Claire, Lily, and I are going to the pool today. I can't wait. I have a brand-new bathing suit that I am excited to wear.

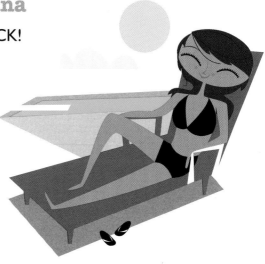

"Mom, can we go now?"

"In a minute."

"Please Mom, we're going to be late."

Finally, we get there. Claire and Lily have already got chairs.
I wave to them and hurry over.

"Hi Claire. Hi Lily."

"Hey Brie. We saved you a chair."

"Thanks!"

I slip my cover-up over my head. Claire is staring at me.

"What?" I ask.

"Uh, nothing."

"Do you like my new suit? I just got it."

"Oh yeah, I do. It's really great."

"Yeah, cool suit Brianna," Lily chimes in.

I spread my towel over the lounge chair and lay out. My
arms are back behind my head. Ahh . . . this is the life. I close
my eyes for a minute and chill out. When I open them, Claire
is staring at me again.

She catches my eye and quickly looks away. What is it? Does
she think my new bathing suit is funny looking? Oh no. Is she
looking at my chest? Do I look too big in a bikini? I start to
ask, but Lily suggests we go swimming.

We have a great time splashing around in the water. After
that we get ice cream. Then it is back to the chairs to warm
up in the sun. Before I know it, our moms are here and it is
time to go home.

"Bye. Call ya later," we say in unison.

When I get home, the first thing I do is go to my room.
I take off my cover-up and look at myself in the mirror. My
bathing suit is cute. It really isn't that different from Claire's.

Everything's all tucked in and covered up. What was she staring at? I can't help it if I'm bigger on top than she is. I hate this.

I raise my arm to brush a stray hair out of my eyes. I see something dark on my armpit. I lift my arm to the mirror for closer inspection. Oh no! There is hair there! That is what Claire was looking at. I am going to die. This is so embarrassing. What should I do? I am never going to wear a bathing suit or anything sleeveless again!

"Mom! Mom!! Where are you?" I yell from my room.

"I'm in my office," she calls back. "If you need me, stop shouting and come to me."

I scramble down the stairs and burst into her office.

"Brie, honey, what's the matter?"

"Um. Nothing."

"Nothing? Then why were you yelling for me?"

"I don't know."

"Was there a problem at the pool?"

"No, not really."

"Did the girls like your new bathing suit?"

"Yea. I think so. They said they did."

"Brianna, what is it? Why are you standing so funny?"

"Mom, I have hair under my arms. It is so gross. I think that Claire totally noticed it, too."

"Oh, I get it. That would make me embarrassed, too. Sweetie, that is perfectly normal for you to grow hair there. Claire will have some one day, too."

"But I hate it. I look like a guy!"

"You do not look like a guy," Mom said with a laugh. "And it is easy enough to get rid of. Come on, let's go into my bathroom and I'll show you how to shave it off."

One of the big responsibilities of puberty is learning to take care of your changing body. Think about all the changes: you have new hair, more sweat and oil, growing parts, and even new smells. Sounds like a lot to handle, but with a little daily attention, you'll be able to keep it under control. Going through puberty means learning to use deodorant, removing unwanted hair, taking care of acne and oily skin, and keeping your body feeling fresh!

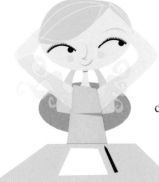

What's That Smell?

Sometime in the beginning of puberty, you or someone close to you will probably notice a new smell coming from your armpits. It's called body odor, and it can be powerful in a not-so-good way. It's one more change caused by those circulating hormones that start the whole puberty thing.

Body odor is pretty easy to handle. The solution is to wash your armpits every day with soap and water. That means you can't just hang out in the shower and sing. You have to raise your arm and soap up under there! After you are clean and dry, it helps to apply deodorant on your pits, too.

There are lots of brands and scents (smells) to choose from. It's hard to find a product that is just a deodorant. Most of them also have an antiperspirant, which makes you sweat less. If your deodorant is not preventing sweat stains on your clothes, try getting one of the "clinical strength" products from your local drugstore.

The best time to apply your deodorant is when you are clean and your pits are dry. If you shower/bathe at night, then it's fine to put your deodorant on at night. Some doctors even think that putting it on at night is best for decreasing sweat the next day. Once a day should be enough, but some girls like to put a little more on in the morning. You'll just have to experiment a little to find out what works best for you.

Your Nose Knows Your Toes!

There's another place that makes some funky smells around puberty time. Yep, your feet can create some major stink. Does your mom put your tennis shoes outside at night? That could be your first clue.

Stinky feet are just another part of puberty. The best way to keep your tootsies fresh is to make sure you wash your feet with soap and water every day, and wear clean cotton socks or footies with any shoes that have closed toes.

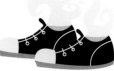

It also helps if you don't wear the same pair of shoes every day. Tennis shoes seem to be the worst, but any shoes can stink. Shoes need some time to air out and let the sweat dry. Giving your favorite pair a day off will pay off!

The Hairy Fairy

In puberty, everyone eventually gets a visit from the hairy fairy. How nice. You may one day notice new hairs in your armpits, darker hair on your legs, and some girls will even get darker hair on their face, especially the upper lip. All this hair is perfectly normal and some girls aren't bothered by it at all. Your ancestors will affect how much hair you grow. And where you live can affect what you do with the hair. In some countries, women don't shave their legs or armpits, and in others, that hair is removed as soon as it shows up. What you do with it will be up to you and your family. We've already mentioned that the pubic hair is there for a reason, and you should probably leave it alone. But what about the rest of the hairy fairy's work?

Hairy Legs and Pits

What about the hair on your legs and in your armpits? It depends on whether it bothers you or not. Girls with blond or light-colored hair may not need to shave at all. Girls with darker hair may want to start sooner. How do you know when it's okay to start shaving or removing that hair? If you feel embarrassed by the hair or if it's starting to bug you, it's probably time to get rid of it.

Hair Be Gone!

There are several ways to remove unwanted hair on your legs and in your pits. There is no one way that works best for everyone, so sometimes you'll just have to try a couple different methods to see which works best for you and your hair.

Here are some of the ways you can get rid of the hair.

Shaving

The most common way girls and women get rid of the hair on their legs and armpits is to shave it off. So, do you just grab your mom's or dad's razor and get to work? No way! It's very important 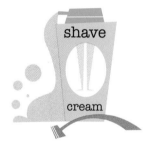 to use your very own razor. Sharing a razor with someone else can spread bacteria and even some pretty bad infections.

In addition to your razor, you'll also need some frothy soap or shaving cream. Make sure the area you are going to shave is wet, then apply the shaving cream or soap until you get a good frothy covering. It takes a little practice to learn how to shave without getting small cuts from the razor, so get some help the first few times.

If you try to shave dry skin, or if you press down too hard with the razor, you can get red, itchy bumps on the area. That's called *razor rash*, and it's no fun! You can prevent razor rash by using a

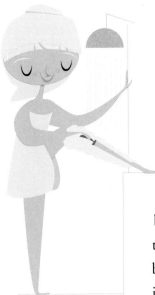

fresh, clean razor, making sure the skin is slick with soapy water or shaving cream, and learning how to hold the razor so you don't have to press down too hard.

Once you start shaving, the hair usually grows back in a few days. When it grows back, it will be stiffer and a little prickly. Some girls only need to shave about once a week, but others need a little more. If you decide to stop shaving, the hair will eventually become softer again and not so prickly, but it takes several weeks, maybe even longer. That's why some moms want you to wait, because once you start shaving, you have to keep shaving pretty regularly to keep your legs smooth, hair-free, and not prickly.

Creams (also called depilatory creams)

There are several types of creams that you can buy that will dissolve the hair off your legs or armpits. Do *not* use these creams on your face unless they say they are especially for faces!

Apply the cream over your legs or armpits and leave on for a certain number of minutes. (The instructions will be on the package.) Use a timer or watch the clock very carefully! When the cream has been on the correct length of time, remove it by rinsing with warm water or using a wet washcloth. Don't scrub the skin too hard or that can cause irritation.

The biggest problem with these creams is that for some girls, the chemicals in the cream are too strong and can cause a rash or irritation. If you want to use a cream hair remover, it's really important to test it on a small area of skin first, and wait a day or two to make sure it doesn't cause a rash or blisters on your skin. If your skin does fine with the test area, then you can use it on the rest of the area.

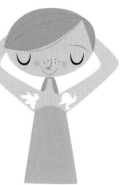

Waxing

To remove hair by "waxing" means that a layer of warm, melted wax is put over the area with unwanted hair. Then a strip of fabric is put over the wax. Last, the fabric is very quickly pulled off and all the hair gets pulled out along with the wax all at once. Ouch is right! But it's very fast and it works well without any irritating chemicals or razor rash. Most of the time, waxing is done by a professional at a salon, but a lot of women learn to wax themselves. If you want to try this at home, you'll definitely need an adult to help so you don't get burned or make a mess! Hair waxing supplies are sold at drugstores and also at beauty supply stores. It's tough to wax hair off your legs because the area is so large, but waxing works really well for smaller areas like your armpits or your upper lip.

Other Hair Removal Methods

There are other ways to remove hair using a laser or electrolysis. These methods are expensive and need to be done by a licensed professional. You may also see ads on TV for special gooey stuff or sandpaperlike things. We're not sure how well those products work, but there are probably easier ways to get rid of a little unwanted hair!

Facial Hair

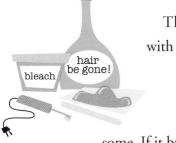

There are some girls, especially those with dark skin and hair, that will grow new hair above their upper lip (in the "mustache" area) as they go through puberty. It may or may not be bothersome. If it bugs you or if it s noticeable, there are a few ways to treat it, but an adult's help is always necessary.

An easy way to make it less noticeable is to lighten the color. There are bleaches for face hair that you can buy at a drugstore. It's important to try the bleach on a small area of skin before using it on your face to make sure you aren't too sensitive or allergic to it. Make sure to follow the directions on the package. When used properly, this can keep the hair nearly invisible for four to six weeks at a time.

If you prefer to remove the hair completely, there are methods that are specifically made for the sensitive skin on the face. The depilatory creams we mentioned above will work on facial hair, but you need to use a product that says it is for face hair. The leg creams can be too harsh for the face. Again, test it on a small area first and follow the directions carefully.

Waxing also works well on facial hair. Other methods like electrolysis and laser treatments are better for older teens and adults. Young skin like yours can be too sensitive for those types of treatments.

Shaving can work, too, but we *don't* recommend using the razor you use on your legs or pits. There are mini-electric razors that have small "heads" made for small areas like your lip. Make sure you have an adult helping if you want to try this method. Some girls worry that shaving will make the hair grow back like man-whiskers. It won't. Facial hairs will grow back a little stiffer, but we promise, you won't get a beard or mustache like a man!

Zits Are the Pits

Along with the hairy fairy, puberty may bring oily skin and pimples, also known as zits or acne. (Gee, thanks!) Acne can start as young as seven years old, but it may get worse during your growth spurt. Some lucky girls never have much of a problem with acne. Others have lots of problems. Once again, thank (or blame) your ancestors.

During puberty, your hormones cause the oil glands in your skin to make more oil. The oil glands are connected to your pores, which are very tiny openings in your skin (you can see them if you look closely).

The oil and cells that line your pores stick together and make a plug that blocks the pore. These plugs are called blackheads.

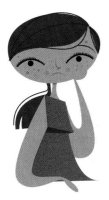

The plug can become a place for lots of skin bacteria to grow. All that bacteria can cause swelling and redness . . . then a pimple is born!

So, acne is *not* caused by dirt alone, but dirt can make it worse. Even the squeakiest clean skin can have acne. Your ancestors also have a lot to do with it. If your parents had acne, you're more likely to have it, too. For help taking care of your skin, see our tips in "Acne Dos and Don'ts" below.

Acne Dos and Don'ts

What Makes Acne Worse?

- ❋ **Picking.** Pinching, picking, and popping your pimples can cause them to become bigger, take longer to heal, or form scars. So no PPPP (pimple pinching, popping, or picking)!

- ❋ **Scrubbing.** Scrubbing too hard with a rough cloth or gritty soaps can be harsh on the skin and make acne worse by irritating pores.

- ❋ **Covering.** Some makeup or cover-ups may clog the pores even more. Make sure you are using oil-free or noncomedogenic products if you feel like you need to try to hide pimples.

- ❋ **Touching.** Certain equipment like helmets or chinstraps can rub the skin and block pores. Even your hands on your face can make acne worse.

* **Stress.** Times of stress (like exams, lack of sleep, lots of worries) can make things worse on your face, and so can your period (we'll talk about that in Chapter 7). Stressful times and periods mean more hormones are being released in your body, and some hormones can make acne worse.

What Makes Acne Better?

* **Washing.** Washing your face twice a day with a mild soap (or acne soap) and warm water should do the trick unless you have those "zit genes." Remember not to scrub. Your hands or a soft washcloth should do the trick.

* **Eating.** Trying to eat a balanced diet is best for your skin. Believe it or not, chocolate, sweets, and French fries don't really make acne worse; they just aren't healthy for you.

* **Exercising.** Regular exercise will increase the blood flow to your skin to give it a healthy glow. The increased blood flow also helps take away the bacteria and germs that make acne worse.

* **Removing.** Try to keep hair products like gel, mousse, oils, or spray off your face and hairline. These products can also block pores.

* **Drinking.** Drinking plenty of water helps keep the skin clear by improving blood circulation and clearing away the bacteria and germs.

If our simple steps for controlling your acne don't work, there are over-the-counter products that can help. Start with the mildest benzoyl peroxide or salicylic acid creams, gels, or face washes, and use small amounts. If you start with a higher strength or use too much, it will cause your skin to get very dry and even peel. This can make the problem worse.

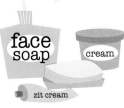

Whatever steps you take, be patient. It takes about six weeks before you'll see the results of a new product or skin care treatment. If that still doesn't do the trick, you may need to see your doctor. There are many treatments that can help.

Taking care of your changing body takes some time to figure out. You may need to try different products, different tricks, and different routines before you find what works best for you and your body. Be patient, and don't be afraid to ask for help if what you're doing isn't working. As you continue to grow, you may need to make changes in the way you take care of yourself. But just make sure you do your best to take *good* care of *you*!

You may need to try different products, different tricks, and different routines before you find what works best for you and your body.

CHAPTER 7

Periods: A Different Kind of Cycle

Riley

"OKAY, RILEY, DINNER IS IN THE FRIDGE. Don't forget to turn off the oven when it's done."

"I know, Mom, you already told me."

"CJ's mom is going to give you a ride to school in the morning. Dad has an early meeting."

"Mom, I know. You've been over all of this. We'll be fine. Have a good trip and don't worry."

"You're right, Riley," Mom says with a smile. "Take care of your father for me."

"I will. No worries."

"Well then this is good-bye. I love you. Take care."

"I love you, too. And I'll see you in a couple of days. Don't worry!"

We hug good-bye and she is off to Toronto. I wish she didn't worry so much. She still thinks that I am a baby.

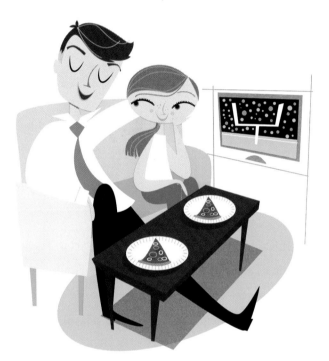

Dad and I eat our dinner in front of the TV so that we can watch the football game. That is a treat! It's kind of fun with just the two of us here. It'd really be perfect if my stomach didn't hurt. I don't say anything to dad. Maybe I just ate too fast. Maybe I just need to go the bathroom.

In the bathroom, I pull down my pants and see BLOOD! I let out the loudest scream of my life. Dad comes running.

"Riley, are you okay? What's the matter?" He asks anxiously.

I try to pull myself together. I am probably dying. I need to keep it together. I am so scared!

"Riley, can you hear me? Are you okay?"

I take a deep breath. "I'm fine."

"What was that scream about? Did you see a mouse?"

I am tempted to say yes. Where is my mom when I need her? But if I am very sick, we should probably go to the doctor. We should probably call an ambulance or a helicopter! I have to tell him. I hope that he doesn't fall apart on me.

I open the door. "Dad, I, uh, well, you see, there's a lot of blood. I think that I may be dying." I try to be brave, but it's no use. I start blubbering. And I never cry. This is bad!

He wraps his arms around me. "Sweetie, I don't think that you are dying."

"You d-d-don't?" I stammer.

"No honey. I think that you have started your period."

"My period?" Oh, I feel so stupid. Why didn't I think of that? It's just that all of that blood was so scary and I didn't expect it.

"Hasn't your mom talked to you about this before?"

"Yeah. And they've talked about it at school. I feel like a dummy."

"You're not a dummy. I'm sure it just came as a surprise. I'm a little surprised, too!"

"I wish Mom was here."

"Me, too, buddy, but we can manage, can't we? Why don't you go take a shower, and I'll see about rounding up some supplies for you."

"Dad, are you sure you know what you are looking for?"

Dad smiles and pats me on the back. "Yes, Riley. I know that we both wish that Mom was here, but dads can handle more than you think."

"I know. I just ... well. Okay. Thanks, Dad."

"Hey, you are going to be all right. I'm proud of my girl. You are becoming a young woman."

"Oh please, Dad. Don't get all weird on me. It's bad enough as it is."

Dad and I watch the rest of the game. I can't help wishing that I were wearing football pads instead of this type of pad. Guess life goes on, ready or not. I'm not sure what I expected, but it really isn't all that bad.

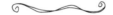

You have probably already heard a little something about periods. And we're not talking about the dot that ends a sentence. The period that happens in puberty is also called *menstruation* or a *menstrual period.* It's a very normal and healthy thing that starts in puberty and continues about once a month until you are close to fifty years old. You'll get your first period a couple of years into puberty, and it's a pretty exciting thing!

The Beginning

When a period starts, there is bloody fluid that comes from the vagina for about three to seven days. That may sound gross and scary, but it is actually an amazing and pretty miraculous event! When you get your period, your body is telling you that you are growing and developing just like you should. It should make you feel good that your body is doing one of the many amazing things it was meant to do.

> It should make you feel good that your body is doing one of the many amazing things it was meant to do.

It's no secret: the whole reason we have periods is so that we can have babies one day if we want to. But having your period won't make you have a baby. It takes a lot more than that. It takes a man *and* a woman to make a baby. That is another big topic. For now, let's stick with puberty and periods.

A period happens because your hormones have told your uterus to get ready for a baby. The uterus gets ready by making a thick, lush "bed" of blood and nutrients inside the uterus. The inside of the uterus has a layer called the *endometrium* (en doe ME tree um) that provides the "bed" for the baby to grow.

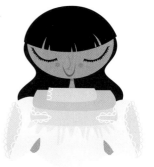

If you think about what we need to survive, it makes sense. To live, all people need shelter, safety, food, water, and oxygen.

Believe it or not, the uterus and endometrium provide exactly this type of environment for a growing baby. The uterus provides the shelter and safe place to grow. The endometrium is lined with nutrients and water. And there is blood that brings oxygen to the baby. What a cool little habitat.

It's a Cycle

Now back to the "bed." If there's no baby, the uterus releases the endometrium. It's sort of like it says, "Oh well, no baby here! It's time to change the sheets." It then releases or sheds the lining of the endometrium, which comes out of the vagina as a period. The whole period contains less than a couple of tablespoons of actual blood. But it seems like more because of the other fluids and tissue that come out with it. Once the uterus sheds the endometrium, it remakes the "bed" with a fresh lining—like fresh sheets—and starts over. This happens about once every month or so. That's why periods are called a cycle.

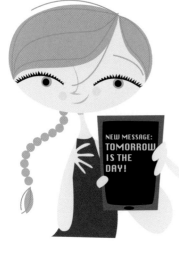

When Will My Period Start!?

Do you think you might get a phone call or a reminder card in the mail to tell you when you'll start your period? Nope. No phone call, no postcard, no text, no IM . . . nothing. There is no way to predict exactly when all this great stuff will happen, but you can use a few clues to guide you. Remember that each girl develops on her own time schedule, so even though you and your friend may have started to develop at the same time, you might start your periods months apart.

Look for these events or times to help you know when you might be close to starting.

* Eighteen to thirty-six months after breast buds

* After growing three or more inches in one year

* When your breasts are in or near Tanner Stage 4

* When your pubic hair reaches Tanner Stage 3 or 4

If you have a chronic medical condition or if you are very athletic or thin, you may start your period later. If you haven't started by age sixteen, you should see your doctor for a checkup to make sure everything is okay.

Your First Period

Your very first period is called *menarche* (MEN are kee). Before menarche, you've already had that vaginal discharge that makes you feel a little wet or damp in your underwear sometimes. In fact, you may not even notice the very moment that your first period starts because you are used to some wetness from your vaginal discharge. When this bloody fluid starts to come out of your vagina, it's only a little to begin with. It's not like someone turns on a faucet or like you have a bad cut. It's usually a little bit more than your discharge. It also may not look exactly like blood. Since it's made of blood, tissue, and other fluids, it can look kind of brown or dark maroon, even blackish.

As we mentioned already, most periods last about three to seven days. It is normal to have a heavier flow of blood in the first couple of days. Then your flow gets lighter toward the end. Occasionally, some girls will bleed longer than that. If your period lasts longer than ten days every month, or if one period lasts longer than two weeks, you should let your doctor know.

Some girls may even have dark clumps of blood called clots. Clots are the consistency of old Jell-O. Clots happen when blood stays in one place for a while—like your vagina. You are most likely to see clots in the morning from the menstrual blood that has been in your vagina while you were lying down.

Your Monthly Visitor

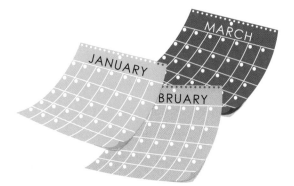

After menarche (your first period), you might have another period about a month later, or it might not come again for several months. In general, girls and women get a period about every month. During your first year, though, it's pretty common for some girls to skip a month or two. Within a year of starting your period, you should expect your periods to happen every 21 to 45 days. If you go more than 90 days between periods, you will want to let your doctor know.

During your first year, though, it's pretty common for some girls to skip a month or two.

Does It Hurt?

For most girls, periods are not painful at all. Some girls will have cramping in their lower abdomen or pelvis before or during their period. Sometimes the pain is even in the vulva, upper thighs, or lower back. This is called menstrual cramping or just "cramps."

Cramps happen because the uterus, which is made of muscle, squeezes to release the endometrial lining that makes up your period. As it squeezes, it can cramp just like any muscle that works hard.

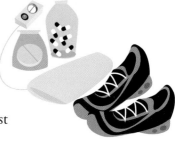

The best treatment for cramping is to exercise, take a warm bath, or use a heating pad. If none of these help, then we recommend taking a medication called ibuprofen or naprosyn. These medications are available at drugstores without a prescription, but you should only take one with permission from a parent or another adult you trust. Follow the directions on the bottle carefully.

There are other products sold at drugstores that claim they are for "premenstrual symptoms" (which means bloating, cramps, and headaches). Interestingly, many of these products contain caffeine, aspirin, and other ingredients that aren't really necessary or as helpful as the medications we mentioned above.

Your Period Is Private, but No Big Secret

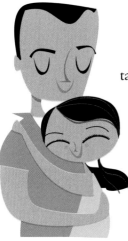

Once you start your period, it's important to tell your mom, and even your dad or another adult you trust. It may seem embarrassing, but remember that all women have periods. And believe it or not, all dads know about periods, too. It's exciting and sometimes a little scary; so don't be afraid to talk with a parent about it.

If you want to keep it private, that's okay, too, but you still should have some way to communicate to a parent about your period, especially because you will need some supplies to help manage it (see the next chapter). Some girls have special names for their period, such as:

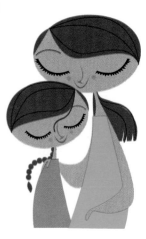

My dot   My monthly

My cousin   Aunt Flo

When you have a special name, you can say to your mom, "Hey Mom, Aunt Flo is visiting." And your mom will know exactly what is going on and can predict how she can help you.

> Having a period doesn't mean you have to act like an adult.

You're Still a Girl!

Getting your period is a big step toward becoming a woman. But guess what? You're still a girl. Having a period doesn't mean you have to act like an adult. Please don't! Keep doing all your great girl things. Dance, play soccer, tumble, run, climb trees, and shoot paintballs. Your period does not have to change any of this.

Even though someone may say, "Oh, you're a woman now," you're not. You're still a girl with lots of great ideas and things to accomplish. Your period doesn't have to slow you down at all!

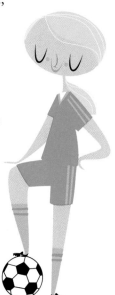

CHAPTER 8

Protective Padding

Lily

I AM SITTING IN MATH CLASS. Mr. Wilson is writing numbers, letters, and symbols on the Smart Board. I hear his voice, but he sounds like the teachers in *Charlie Brown*. "Blah, Bluh, Blah, Bluh, Blah," he drones. I cannot concentrate. I stare at the hands on the clock instead. They seem to be moving in slow motion. We have been sitting here for twenty minutes and have thirty minutes more until class is over. There is no way I am going to make it.

I fidget with my book and my pencil. My foot is tapping on the floor. I cannot keep still, but I cannot move either. What am I going to do? I have my period and I need to change my pad. I thought that I could wait until after class. Now I don't think so. I can't decide which would be more embarrassing—getting up in the middle of class to go to the bathroom with my purse or risking a stain on my pants if I don't. When I consider it this way, my choice is clear.

Mr. Wilson stops talking for a moment and is looking around the class. I decide that now is my time. I raise my hand.

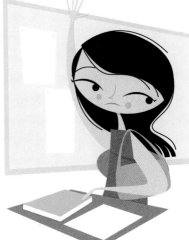

"Yes, Lily. What is the answer?"

"The, uh, answer," I stammer. Was he asking a question? I wasn't paying attention. "Um, well, I don't know." There are some chuckles and snickers around the room. I feel the color rise in my face.

"If you don't know the answer, why did you raise your hand?"

"Why did I raise my hand?" I stupidly repeat. More laughter.

Mr. Wilson takes a deep breath. He moves a step closer toward my desk. Now I am wondering if I might just faint.

"I need to use the restroom," I blurt out. Before he can say another word, I grab my purse and dart for the door. I feel every eye on me. It feels like a nightmare.

I go to the bathroom, change my pad, and wash my hands. I splash some water on my face and try to calm down. The door opens and there is Claire. I run over to her and give her a hug.

"I am so embarrassed! I don't want to go back to class."

"No one has any idea what was going on," says Claire. "Now come on back to class. It will be fine. Just smile and act like nothing happened. Besides, you're Mr. Wilson's best student. He could never be upset with you."

"Are you sure?" I ask.

"Positive," Claire says with a smile.

"Okay," I agree. I wait for Claire to come with me.

"You better go ahead, so he doesn't think that I went to the bathroom just to see you."

"But you did!" I say.

"I know that, and you know that, but he doesn't have to know that!"

I start to open the door to the hallway, and then I stop. "Thanks Claire. You are the best!"

"I know," she laughs.

My hand starts to shake a bit as I walk back into math class. I am smiling, though, thinking of Claire. I walk back to my desk. Everyone is working on a problem. A couple of heads pop up briefly, and then return to their work. I sit back down and sigh. Phew! Claire was right. No big deal.

Have you ever seen the aisle at the grocery store that has all the "feminine hygiene products" in it? You know the one . . . it has lots and lots of pastel-colored boxes and mostly women in the aisle? Sometimes there are hundreds of different types of products. Why so many? It all has to do with periods. Every girl and woman has different likes and dislikes when it comes to taking care of their flow.

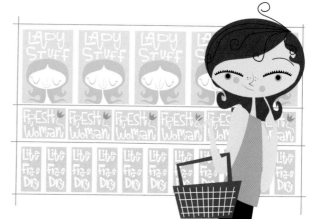

Of course, you will need to "take care of your flow," too. If you don't, you'll end up with blood on your clothes and bedsheets. That would just be too messy. Those "feminine products" are specifically made for managing menstrual flow and protecting your clothes. And there are tons of different brands in tons of different shapes and sizes. After a period or two, you'll figure out which ones work best for you.

Pads

Most girls prefer to use a "pad" with their first period. A pad, also called a sanitary napkin (who came up with that horrible name?), is an oval or rectangular cottony pad that fits in your underwear and absorbs the menstrual blood as it comes out. Pads are made with an adhesive strip that holds them in the crotch of your underwear. Just unwrap the pad, pull off the paper that covers the adhesive strip, and put the pad in your underwear. The sticky side goes against your underwear, *not* against *you*!! (Ouch!) As you pull up your underwear, you'll want to make sure the pad is positioned so it is centered below your vagina. If it is too far forward or backward, it might miss some of the flow.

Pads with "Wings"

Pads with "wings" were invented to help prevent the leaking and overflow that may happen when a pad bunches up in the middle. Sometimes a lot of 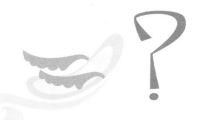 running or other physical activity will make your pad bunch up so that your menstrual flow goes over the edge and stains your underwear. Wings are extra flaps with their own adhesive strips that wrap around the crotch of your underwear. This keeps the blood from getting on the edges of the crotch part of your underwear. Some girls like wings. Some don't. Most types of pads come with or without wings. Your choice.

Choosing a Pad

Just like girls come in different sizes and shapes, there are pads in different sizes and shapes to match your body type. There are shorter pads for petite girls and longer pads for bigger or taller girls. And then, there are the minis, the maxis, the supers, and the lights. How's a girl to choose? You'll just have to try a few to find your favorite. Here is a list of some of the types you'll find in that special aisle.

- **Panty liners.** These are really thin pads that work for very light bleeding—like you'll have toward the end of your period. Some girls also like to use these for the vaginal discharge they have between periods.

- **Minipads or "light" pads.** These pads are a little thicker than a panty liner. They are best for light to normal menstrual flow.

- **Maxipads or Super pads.** Maxi pads are fluffy and big, and they can feel pretty thick. But they sure come in handy when your period is the heaviest.

- **Overnight pads.** As you can imagine, when you lie down your flow can run in different directions. Overnight pads are longer and bigger to help cover a larger "area" while you sleep. Some girls just use a regular pad at night. It depends on you and your flow.

- **Reusable pads.** For the environmentally conscious girl, reusable pads are made of cotton and are washable. They are better for the environment because they can be washed and reused. They may be hard to find, but most health food or natural food stores carry them. They are also available through catalogs and online.

Besides choosing from all these different shapes and sizes, you'll also have to choose between deodorized and nondeodorized pads. Deodorized pads have a perfumelike smell to them. When menstrual blood mixes with sweat, it can have an odor. But if you bathe with soap and water daily, especially during your period, you won't need to worry about menstrual odor. There is no smell that anyone would be able to notice. If you feel more comfortable using deodorized pads—go ahead. But some girls get skin irritations or itching from the perfumes in the pads.

Speaking of odor, the other things you might see in the "feminine hygiene" aisle are special "feminine deodorant" sprays. They are made to be sprayed "down there," but they are totally not necessary. We're not sure who decided that a vagina should smell like a flower, but it really doesn't and it shouldn't. As long as you wash daily, there is no need for these sprays or perfumes, especially in the sensitive vulva area.

How Long Do Pads Last?

You already know your period will last three to seven days. Pads only last three to seven *hours* depending on your flow. Your pad probably will never be completely covered in blood, but once the center part gets pretty full, it's time to change it. Also, don't wear the pad so long that it starts to feel soaked or soggy. Pads are made to pull the moisture away from your skin. When your pad starts to feel wet or smushy, you will also know that it is time to change it.

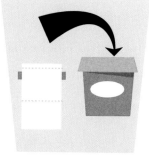

So, when your pad is full, do you just pull it off and flush it down the toilet? Please don't! Pads will totally clog a toilet or cause it to back up and overflow. Embarrassing, and not good for the plumbing!

Well then, do you just plop it in the trash can or leave it on the floor for everyone to see? Not! Nobody wants to look at your used pads. When you are changing a pad, just wrap it in toilet paper or the wrapper from the new pad you are putting on,

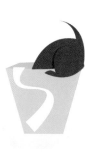

and put it in the trash can. At home, you should have a trash can near your toilet. You should also get in the habit of emptying your own trash can when it has used pads in it. In time, they will start to smell bad. Got a dog? Take the trash out even more often! It can be really

embarrassing to have your dog prancing around with your used
pad in his mouth . . . yuck!

By cleaning up after
yourself, you are
showing responsibility.

At school or out in public, most bathroom stalls have a special small trash container on the stall wall for used pads. Ahhh! So that's what it's for! You thought it was for used gum, didn't you? Now you know. By cleaning up after yourself, you are showing responsibility. This is one of those growing-up things that shows you are taking care of yourself and your body.

Tips for Period Troubles

Having a period will present some new challenges and even
some frustrations for you sometimes. Here are some tips that
might help make things a little easier.

While you sleep. If you're a wild sleeper or have a heavy
flow, it can help to place a towel under you at night in
case you soak through or spill over your pad. That way
you can just wash the towel instead of all your bed sheets.

Stains. If you get blood on your clothes or sheets (and you
will), wash them as soon as you can and use cold water
and soap. Hot water can make blood stains harder to get
out. A brief washing by hand can get most of the stain
out. The rest will usually come out in the laundry.

Tough stains! If you have a large or heavy stain that is tough to get out, a mild chemical called hydrogen peroxide (you can buy it in a pharmacy store) can help dissolve the blood. Ask a grown-up for help using it because it can change or fade the color of some fabrics. If you have a big mess, get help! Don't use spray spot removers or bleach directly on the crotch of your underwear. These are harsh chemicals that can cause a lot of irritation to the skin of your vulva and vagina.

No pads. If you start your period and don't have a pad handy, you can put some toilet paper in your underwear and head to the school nurse's office, to your backpack, or to your best friend for a pad. Toilet paper won't work for long because it tends to "wander" in your underwear.

Leaks. If your clothing is stained, first ask a friend if the stain is visible. A lot of period stains look horrible to you, but people behind you can't even see them! If it's visible, try to find a sweater or jacket to tie around your waist until you can get a change of clothes.

Most girls choose to use pads with their first period. Sometimes, though, a pad just won't do the job you need it to do. Read on to learn about other options for managing your *menses* (that means periods!).

CHAPTER 9

Things with Strings (Tampons!)

Riley

I AM IN THE RESTROOM AT SCHOOL washing my hands when I hear moaning coming from one of the stalls. Then I hear a loud sob and some sniffling. Someone is crying. Should I stay and try to help or leave so that she is not embarrassed? Before I can decide, the stall door opens and out comes Tess. She opens her red-rimmed eyes wide and lets out a gasp.

"Riley, what are you doing?" she demands.

I'm about to apologize, when I stop myself. I've done nothing wrong. This is the same girl who made fun of me. This is the same girl who treats everyone like dirt. I will not let her intimidate me.

"Nothing, just washing my hands," I reply with a voice stronger than I feel.

"Oh," Tess whispers quietly. "I'm sorry. I didn't mean to yell at you. I'm just having a really bad day."

What? Did Tess apologize to me? Am I in some sort of alternate universe?

She splashes water on her face. I turn to leave. She looks so pitiful. I can't go.

"What's the matter?" I ask.

"The big swim meet is today and I can't ..." She starts to cry again.

"Tess, you are the best swimmer in the school. You are going to do great."

"I know, but I can't swim in it."

Well, she's still as confident as ever. Wonder why she can't do the meet.

"Why not?" I ask.

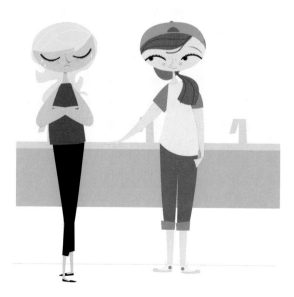

"I just can't, okay?" she replies.

"Okay," I say. I start for the door.

"Riley, wait. I know that we are not the best of friends, but I really need someone to talk to."

Understatement of the year, I think, but I say, "All right."

"The thing is, I, uh, started my period," Tess says.

"I don't understand. Why can't you swim?"

"Why can't I swim? Didn't you hear me? I started my *period!*"

"I did hear you, but you can still swim. Just use a tampon."

"A tampon?"

"Yes. I'm sure that your mom has some. She can help you after school. The meet's not until tonight, right?"

"Yeah. I don't know. That seems like totally embarrassing."

"Come on, it's your mom. Besides, it couldn't be more embarrassing than explaining why you are missing the meet?"

"Well, no. I guess I could try it," Tess says with a shrug.

"Okay. Good luck."

"Hey Riley, thanks, and please don't mention this to anyone."

"You're welcome, Tess, and don't worry. I won't."

Claire catches up with me as I leave the restroom.

"What took you so long?" she asks.

"I wasn't that long. Hey, what's for lunch? I'm starved!"

"I'm not sure, but I'm starved, too. Let's go."

I'm not going to tell anyone about Tess. What is it they are always telling us? Treat others as you would like to be treated. Wish that Tess would learn that lesson, but at least I know that she is slightly more human than I thought.

Have you ever looked at a tampon? I mean, actually tore the wrapper off one and examined it. Go ahead, we'll wait . . . we bet there's a box under a bathroom sink somewhere in your house. A tampon is kind of funny looking, made of stiff cotton and plastic or cardboard, with a string hanging out one end. At a glance, it doesn't look like it's good for much. There was a scene in a movie where a boy used one to stop a nose bleed. That might work, but the truth is that tampons can really help you manage your periods.

A tampon is a small, cylinder-shaped cotton "tube" that actually fits inside the vagina and absorbs the menstrual flow as it comes out of the cervix (the cervix is the opening to your uterus at the top of your vagina). This may sound painful, but really, if a tampon is put in correctly, you won't even feel it.

Why on earth would you want to use a tampon? Tampons are nice because you can swim or do other activities without having to worry about a bulky pad. Can you imagine trying to wear a pad with your bathing suit, then getting it wet in the pool? (Have you ever seen a soaked swimmie diaper?) No thanks. For swimmers, dancers, and gymnasts, tampons are sometimes a necessity. For everyone else, it just depends on your preference. Some girls never want to use a tampon, and other girls can't imagine having a period without using tampons. It's all about what you prefer.

> Some girls never want to use a tampon, and other girls can't imagine having a period without using tampons.

What if you are an ace swimmer, like Tess, and you start your period the day before a huge meet? Do you have to skip the meet? No way. You can use a tampon with your very first period if you want. Your period doesn't need to stop you from doing any of your activities.

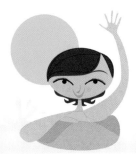

If you don't have a big swim meet or other "emergency" need for a tampon, most girls like to try their first tampon after they have had a few periods.

How to Use a Tampon

Tampons are put into your vagina using something called an applicator. An applicator is made of smooth cardboard or plastic and helps you slide the tampon into your vagina. The first time you use one, you may need help from your mom or big sister or even a friend who has used one. Some girls do fine by themselves after reading the instructions. A mirror can help, too.

the tampon is inside here!

——applicator

—— gripper groves

—plunger

—string

It sounds scary to put something in your vagina, but once you learn how to use a tampon, it's easy! First you need to know the parts of the tampon. (See the illustration.) They are the applicator, the tampon, the string, the plunger—and the grooves for holding it. Then follow these steps.

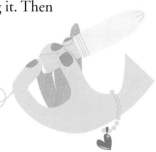

1. Find a position that lets you comfortably reach your vagina. You may want to sit on the toilet, squat, or lie down.

2. Do your best to relax!

3. Unwrap the tampon and hold it on the "gripper grooves" with the string hanging down.

4. Find your vaginal opening using a mirror or your finger.

5. Hold the tampon between your thumb and middle finger like this:

6. Insert the tampon gently into your vagina and aim it toward your lower back. That's the normal angle of the vagina.

7. Push it in until your fingers touch your vulva.

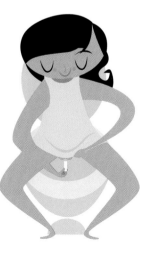

8. Push the plunger all the way in (you can push the plunger with the pointer finger on the same hand, or use your other hand to help).

9. Pull the applicator out.

10. Your tampon will be in the vagina and the string will be on the outside. Ta da!

You'll know if you have the tampon in correctly by the way it feels. If you can't feel it, it's in right. If it's uncomfortable and makes you want to waddle when you walk, you didn't get it far enough into your vagina. You can either use your finger to push it in higher, or pull it out and start over with a new tampon.

All tampons have a string on them. To get the tampon out, you just pull slowly but firmly on the string. Don't worry: the string won't break. Even if it did, the vagina is sort of a "dead end," so a tampon cannot get lost inside your body.

Should I Practice for the Big Day?

Does all this information make you want to practice for the big day? No way! There's no need to practice, but it's fine to open up a tampon and see what it looks like. You can even plunk it in a glass of water to see what happens to it. But using a tampon when you are not having a period is *not* a good idea! If you're not having your period, there won't be enough fluid in your vagina to wet the tampon. The tampon needs to be wet with your menstrual flow before you take it out. Taking out a dry tampon pulls on the vagina too much and can hurt.

Choosing the Right Tampon

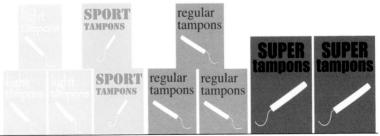

As you might expect, there are different sizes and shapes of tampons—just like there are pads! The first time you use one, try a slender or "light" size. These are thinner and smaller than regular or super tampons. That makes them more comfortable to use until you are better at getting them in and taking them out.

The light tampons are for lighter flows. The regulars are for normal flow. And the super and super-plus are for really heavy flows. They all will fit in a normal vagina, but it's always easier to start with the smallest ones.

If you use tampons, there is no need for deodorized tampons (even through you'll see them on the shelves in the store). Blood has no odor while it is inside the vagina. With tampons, the blood stays in the vagina on the tampon until you change it. The deodorized tampons are pretty useless and the perfumes used on them can be irritating for some girls.

When to Change Your Tampon?

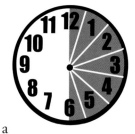

You can't look at a tampon to see when it is getting full (because it is inside you). Instead, you have to judge by the way it feels, or just change your tampons regularly. When a tampon gets full, the menstrual flow will soak the string and even leak out onto your underwear. For that reason, some girls like to wear a minipad along with a tampon until they are more confident using them.

You should never wear a tampon for more than six hours. If you're using the right size for your flow, most will only last about four hours. We don't recommend using them at night while you sleep. In your groggy morning routing, you might forget you have one in there and forget to take it out. And if you're getting the sleep you really need, it would be in longer than six hours. And that's too long!

Are Tampons Dangerous?

Some people worry about an infection called toxic shock syndrome (TSS) that has been caused by tampon use. This was a more common problem years ago and mostly happened with a certain type of tampon that is no longer made. Toxic shock syndrome is caused by one type of bacteria, and it is very rare. Millions of women use tampons every day without getting TSS. If you change your tampons regularly, there's no need to worry about TSS.

To Flush or Not to Flush: Tampon Disposal

Like with pads, you'll need to be responsible when you use tampons. When you remove a tampon, it's best to wrap it up and throw it in the trash. Tampons can be flushed, but

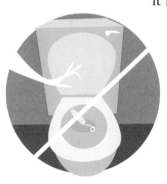

it is best not to because some toilets (especially newer ones) get clogged even by small tampons. Some applicators are supposed to be flushable, too, but it's best to just throw those away as well (and it's polite to wrap them up also). Be kind to your plumbing (and keep the plumbers away)!

Wrapping Things Up ...

Besides learning to wrap up your pads and tampons, we want to wrap up this chapter by letting you know that having a period is as normal as growing breasts. Even though it feels awkward at first, you'll get used to it and it will be just one more part of who you are and what you do. Don't forget that you may need help from your mom or even your dad when it comes to managing your period and other girl things.

For more information on periods and details on period problems, check out the next *Girlology* book, called *Girlology: A Girl's Guide to Stuff That Matters.*

CHAPTER 10

Growing a Strong and Healthy Body

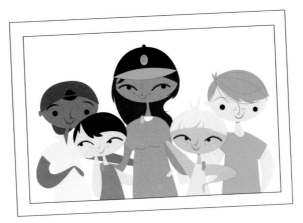

Brianna

MRS. HARRIS IS LINING US UP for our class picture.
Claire is front and center. Lily and Riley are in the row behind
her. Me? I am in the back row, of course. I am the tallest girl in
the class. Taller than just about all the boys. Mrs. Harris tells us
to "Smile!" Argh. I don't really feel like smiling.

Lately, my height seems like everyone's favorite topic of conversation. There are the "lend me a hand" comments. "Hey Brianna, can you reach that book for me?" or "Brie, would you mind getting the crystal bowl down for me?" That one's from my mom, who is a good four inches shorter than me. Then there are the surprised and "can't believe" comments. "My goodness, look at what a big girl you are!" Or "Every time I see you you've grown another inch." Or simply, "I can't believe how *tall* you are!" My least favorite comments about my height are the silent ones. They are made with the eyes. Eyes that grow wide as they take in all of me. And even though their eyes are clearly marveling at how high I extend from the ground, they make me feel very small inside.

The only time that I truly relax and put my height out of mind is when I am running. I love to run. I forget all of my worries and just let go. I feel free. I feel light and happy. And I feel fast. And not to brag, but I am fast. I run for our school's varsity track team. This weekend we are headed to the state championships. The school has never won before. Coach thinks that I will make a big difference.

After practice, I walk home. I open the door and smell Mom's lasagna. Yum! I'm starved. I head straight to the kitchen. My Aunt Terry is there. I forgot that she was coming to visit. Before I can even say hello, she has her arms around me in a big hug.

"Look at you! Would you just look at you?" she exclaims.

I wait because I know what is coming next, something about how big or grown-up or tall I am. Then she pulls back and looks and smiles real big and says, "Brianna, honey, you are truly beautiful! I am so glad to see you."

I smile back at her and remember why she is my favorite aunt. We sit around the table and eat the delicious lasagna. My dad starts bragging about me and track and the championships. Aunt Terry says that she is probably more excited than he is about the competition. Now I find that hard to believe!

Two days later we travel an hour to compete. I run the 400 and the 800. I am the youngest one in the race today. Some of these girls have driver's licenses and boyfriends! Right before the race, Aunt Terry pulls me aside and gives me a lucky coin to put in my running shoe. Then she says, "Just stretch those legs of yours as far as you can and have fun."

I can't feel the coin, it is so thin, but I know it is there. I can feel my heart. I think that it is beating so hard it just might beat through my skin! I run as I hard as I can. I stretch my legs, as Aunt Terry said, and I push myself. I come in second in the 400, but I win the 800! I even set a new record. Best of all, our school wins the state championship! I am beyond excited. They place a red, white, and blue ribbon with a medal on it around my neck. It feels wonderful. Then they line us up for a picture. This time when the photographer says "Smile!"—I do. I really smile.

My family practically attacks me with hugs and praise. Dad says, "You are just like your Aunt Terry!" I had forgotten that Aunt Terry used to run track too. She is almost as tall as my dad. She puts her arm around me and says, "Don't you just love being tall?"

I answer, "You know what? I do! I love being tall."

If puberty is all about "growing" into an adult body, then there's a lot more to it than just breasts and hair, right? There's that part about getting taller and bigger. That's the part that really starts to amaze the adults in your life. One day you are a miniperson always looking up at the adults around you, and within six months to a year, all your pants are too short and you are actually looking eye-to-eye with adults. It's yet another amazing accomplishment of puberty.

It's not like you haven't been growing and suddenly, in puberty, you do. It's just that you've never grown so fast! That's why it can hurt sometimes. (Yes, growing pains are real!) Remember that the puberty growth spurt starts with your hands and feet. Then your arms and legs grow. The year before your period starts, you might even grow several inches or more!

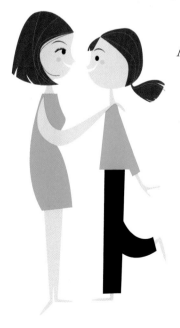

Body Up and Out

And you aren't just growing up. There are times where you grow "out" more than you grow "up." Your whole shape is changing and becoming curvier. Your hips will grow out, your waist may be more obvious, your rear may get bigger, and your breasts are definitely growing out. All this growth during puberty can be frustrating because once you get used to a change (and have clothes that fit you well), more change happens! But there is a point where it all slows down and you can wear the same size clothes for a long time. In fact, once your period starts, your growth slows down a lot, even though it will continue a little for a few more years.

Watch Your Step!

While you are growing so fast, you may feel clumsy or awkward. Your bones are growing faster than your muscles. While your muscles are catching up, they don't work as well as usual. So, if you play sports or do activities that require balance and coordination, you may have some "off" times during your growth. You may stumble, have trouble with balance, or just not have the same moves that you've always had. Be patient! Keep practicing! Once your muscles catch up with your bones and have a chance to adjust, you'll be even better than you were before you grew!

Growing Is Hard Work

It may not seem like it, but growing is hard work for your body. In order to grow well, your body needs to be fed well, exercised well, and rested well. This is the most important time to develop healthy habits. Believe it or not, the healthy habits you start now can help you through the rest of your life. Unhealthy habits (like trying to live on chocolate, ice cream, and potato chips, or letting your computer keyboard provide your only exercise) are hard to break! Healthy habits can even help you live longer! So now is a great time to make a promise to yourself to focus on eating foods that are healthy, getting regular exercise, and getting enough sleep. That way all your growing will give you a new look that looks and feels great on you!

Here are some simple tips for a healthier you:

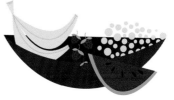

* Never skip breakfast!
* Eat small but healthy snacks between meals
* Don't forget 5 to 6 servings of fruits and veggies every day (the more color on your plate, the better!)
* Let "sweets" be special treats, not a daily habit
* Drink 6 to 8 glasses of water every day (really!)

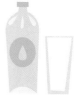

* Stay away from soda and any drink that lists a type of "syrup" or "sugar" as one of the first few ingredients on the label
* Exercise for at least one hour every day (it doesn't have to be all at once)

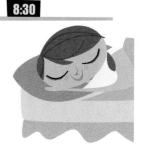

* Sleep at least 8 to 9 hours every night (too little sleep can slow down your thinking and make you grumpy, hungry, and weak!)

Treat It Well!

All this growing and changing can leave you feeling confused or downright unhappy with the way your body looks. What's most important to remember is that your body will continue to change. Most of these changes will help you accomplish amazing things, but you have to continue to take care of your body with healthy eating and drinking, exercise, and rest.

The coolest thing about growing and about this time of your life is that you will be able to do so many new things that make it clear you are not a little kid anymore. You are becoming stronger, smarter, and better at complicated stuff. There are some girls your age who can do back flips, score soccer goals, write a song, run a 5K race, jump a horse, paint a landscape, do a triple Lutz, climb a mountain, or skate a half-pipe. If you treat your body well and appreciate all that it can do for you, you may be surprised by how awesome it can be!

Before you know it, you are growing, growing, then GROWN!

CHAPTER 11

True-Blue Friends

Claire

I AM STANDING BY THE LOCKERS with Lily and Brianna. We are planning to get together to study for our big geography test. Riley walks up to us. She kind of stands there chewing on her lip like she wants to say something.

I say, "Hi Riley. I like your shirt. Is it new?" She is wearing a purple, cotton blouse with a ruffle neckline and sleeves. Very cute and girly. Not at all like the T-shirts Riley normally wears.

"Hi Claire. Thanks! It is new. You don't think it looks stupid?"

"Are you kidding? You look great!" I say. Then Lily and Brianna chime in. "Hey Riley, cute top," says Lily.

"Love it," adds Brianna.

Riley is really beaming now. "Thanks so much. Well, guess I'll be going now. Need to study for geography."

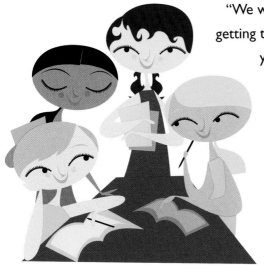

"We were just talking about getting together to study. Do you want to come?" asks Brianna.

"That would be great!" exclaims Riley. Then she pauses, "Are you sure you don't mind?"

"Don't be silly. The more the merrier," I say. "Why doesn't everyone meet at my house at four?"

A couple of hours later we are all gathered in my bedroom. We are sitting on the floor with our books and notes scattered in between us. The test is on Europe. We need to know all of the countries, their locations, and their capitals. Brianna is pretending to be a game show host and quizzing us on the capitals. She alternates between a British and a French accent. We are laughing so hard, tears are streaming down our faces.

"Last question," she says in her clipped, fake British voice. "Who can tell us the capital of Belarus?"

Lily's hand shoots up.

"Minsk," Lily says with authority.

"You are correct!" British Brianna declares. "You have won 200,000 pounds!"

We all whoop and cheer in delight.

"Hey, let's take a study break. I think that we've earned it!"
I say. We sit around and talk for a while. Then Lily spots some
of my teen magazines. We ooh and aah over our celebrity
crushes. Then we spot a quiz. It is entitled, "What Kind of
Friend Are You: True Blue, Lukewarm, or Screamin' Not?"
(See the quiz on page 120.)

"Let's take it!" says Brianna.

We read the questions and laugh at the "b" answers. As if
any of us would act that way. We are somewhat divided over
whether to pick "a" or "c."

"I could see picking 'a' sometimes," I say.

"Me, too," adds Riley. "I don't like to embarrass people, and
talking about deodorants is totally embarrassing!"

"Wait a minute! Are you saying that you would rather smell
bad then talk about smelling bad?" asks Brianna.

"Maybe," answers Riley.

"I think a real friend is someone that cares enough to tell
you the truth, even when it's not easy." Lily looks at each of us
as she speaks. All four of us should make a pact right here and
now to be "True-Blue Friends."

I have to admit Lily is right, but I don't have to admit it out
loud. We take the quiz and average all of our points and . . .
together we are True-Blue Friends!

What Kind of Friend Are You

True Blue, Lukewarm, or Screamin' Not?

1. You notice your friend has something yucky stuck in her teeth, you—

    ❑ a. Say nothing and try not to look at her mouth.

    ❑ b. Scream in horror, point to her teeth, and say, "Ew, gross!"

    ❑ c. Quietly point to your own teeth and mouth, "You have a little something stuck right there."

2. Your friend hs a giant pimple smack dab in the middle of her forehead. You—

    ❑ a. Say nothing. You ignore her pimple and ignore her.

    ❑ b. Scream in horror, point to her forehead, and say, "OMG! That is the biggest zit I've ever seen!"

    ❑ c. Ignoring the zit, but not her, you compliment her outfit.

3. You notice your friend has a bad case of B.O. You—

    ❑ a. Say nothing and stay clear.

    ❑ b. Scream in horror, wave your hands over your nose, and say, "You stink!"

    ❑ c. Try to start a conversation about your favorite deodorant.

4. Your friend has big time bad breath. You—

    ❑ a. Say nothing and move a little farther away.